SMO2004972
19-5-03
£17.99

GG
(ha)

# Learning Journals a
## Incidents: *Reflective*
## *health care professionals*

1856421538

# Key Management Skills in Nursing

**Other books in the series**

Key management Skills in Nursing
Edited by Roswyn A Brown and George Castledine

# Learning Journals and Critical Incidents: *Reflective practice for health care professionals*

*by*
*Tony Ghaye and Sue Lillyman*

Quay
Books

Quay Books Division, Mark Allen Publishing Ltd
Jesses Farm, Snow Hill, Dinton, Nr Salisbury, Wiltshire, SP3 5HN

© Mark Allen Publishing Ltd 1997
First reprint 1999
Second reprint 2001
Third reprint 2003

ISBN 1 85642 153 8

British Library Cataloguing-in-Publication Data
A catalogue record is available for this book

Printed in the UK by Biddles Limited, Guildford, Surrey

# Contents

# Foreword

*'If the public is to trust nurses to use their knowledge and skill to act at all times in their* (patients, clients, residents) *best interests... Nurses, like all health professionals, must monitor and update their standards of conduct so that they can be held accountable.'*

(George Castledine, 1996)

This statement and many others of the same ilk, are centrally about competent and confident clinical practice. The knowledge, skills and sensitivities required can be derived from many sources and in different ways. For example, the knowledge can be personal and practical. The skills can be psychomotor, social or cognitive. The sensitivities associated with perceptions of dignity, compassion, rights and morality. Additionally all health care professionals act in a context, for example in small or larger teams, within an NHS Trust or the community. The context for care is influenced and bounded by people, places and things, all of which are linked and interact in particular ways to try to serve the public interest and the common good.

This book is intended to support health care professionals in becoming more personally and publically accountable. It is therefore educative in its intent in that it tries to help all health care professionals to reflect on what may well be perceived as competent and skilful clinical action. Through the more generic process of reflective practice and the more specific and related approaches of journal writing and critical incident analysis, we hope that health care professionals may be able to make even more sense of their clinical worlds by additionally inquiring into, and understanding more richly, that which is often implicit in everyday practice. In doing so the book takes the reader into a health care landscape which is intellectual, emotional, moral and ethical. Issues of power, politics, interests and truth need to be confronted. We invite you to interact with the text in the spirit of lifelong learning and managing for quality.

Tony Ghaye and Sue Lillyman
March, 1997

## References

Castledine G (1996) Setting new ethical standards for practice is a collaborative process. *BJN* **5** (4): 256

# Acknowledgements

In constructing this book we acknowledge our debt of thanks for the support and stimulating dialogues we have had with our colleagues who have encouraged us to write a book of this kind. In particular, we thank our students on the portfolio development course in Birmingham, the ENB 997/998 courses in Hereford, Worcester and Kidderminster, Teresa Lehane for her inspirational work with children with profound and multiple learning difficulties, Liz Fradd, Gill Wilkins, Maggie Goodchild, Margaret Taylor, Marion Taylor, Julie Cadle, Fred Soobhany, Linda Dunn and Kay Danai.

## Dedication

To our parents: Marjorie and John, Jean and Reg

# Introduction

This book is designed to assist health care professionals to develop the art of learning from reflective practice. Journal writing and the analysis of critical incidents are two of the ways to facilitate reflection. Specifically they relate to the art of reflection-on-action. This is reflection which takes place after an event and often out of the clinical area.

Reflection is a means of learning from and improving practice (Street, 1991). Just as the process of health care itself continuously unfurls, so too does reflective practice. Reflection-on-action focuses upon who we are, what we know and what we can do with this to improve the quality of the care we can give.

The book is divided into three broad sections to do with 'context', 'learning processes' and 'outcomes'. In **Section A: Context**, the genesis, goals and interests of reflective practice are set out. Although the art of reflective practice has been formally introduced into the health care arena via the 'Post Registration and Practice' (PREP) requirements (UKCC, 1992) and the government's 'Vision for the Future' (DOH, 1993) it is not a new idea and is traced back to Dewey at the turn of the twentieth century. Following on from this we look at the way a variety of writers have organised the processes of learning through reflection into 'models'. A number of models are critiqued and then organised into a typology. Taken together the two chapters in the first section remind us that it is difficult to know what we cannot see. The four chapters in the second section give us two lenses to do just this.

**Section B: Processes** describes and justifies journal writing and critical incident analysis as two ways to learn from reflection-on-action. Examples of each process, drawn from clinical practice, are given. Learning through journal writing and the analysis of critical incidents gives weight to the idea that we should not assume that clinical practice is naturally self-disclosing. It often does not speak for itself. It is not always transparent and familiar. The examples we present and interrogate make the point that the value, significance and meaning of our clinical practice has to be constructed and interpreted. These constructions are historically, politically, economically, socially and culturally determined.

In the final section, **Outcomes** we take a look at some of the implications for clinical practice that arise from reflecting-on-action through journal writing and critical incident analysis. These processes are appropriate to all health care professionals at any stage of their career. It is through reflection-on-action that individual practitioners and groups of health care professionals generate opportunities to nourish their practice and improve the quality of the care they provide to their client group.

# References

Department of Health (1993) *A Vision for the Future, The Nursing, Midwifery and Health Visiting Contribution to Health and Health Care*

Street A (1991) *From Image to Action: Reflection in nursing practice.* Deakin University Press, Melbourne

UKCC (1992) *Post Registration and Practice.*UKCC, London

# Section A:
# Context

# 1

# Reflective practice in perspective

## Introduction

In recent years reflection and reflective practice have become well known words within the health care arena. They are words that have been debated and discussed within the clinical environment, nursing literature and have recently become a part of every nurse's, health visitor's and midwife's vocabulary.

This chapter will attempt to identify where these terms and concepts originated from and their place within clinical practice today. It will attempt to identify how they can be used as evidence of personal and professional development. It will also attempt to demystify some of the interpretations that writers have given to the area of reflection and reflective practice. These interpretations have caused some confusion and are partially responsible for some of the resistance to these concepts being implemented in clinical practice.

Finally, it will attempt to discuss how the individual practitioner can apply these processes to their clinical practice, identifying how to provide evidence of their professional development in line with the PREP (UKCC, 1990) requirements utilising the skills for their own development.

## Historical perspective

Reflection and reflective practice are not new ideas that have recently been identified to complicate the practitioner's life, nor are they unique to the health care arena. Many other professional groups are familiar with the principles and procedures of reflective practice. These include the teaching profession, police training and other allied health care professionals.

It was Dewey in 1933 who initially defined reflective practice in his work. Over time many others have given their definitions including Mead (1934), Mezirow (1981), Schon (1987), Johns (1994), Burnard (1995) and Ghaye *et al* (1996). All the writers on this subject have set out their conceptions in a slightly different way. These multiple interpretations have partially led to the confusion that surrounds the terms today.

It is claimed that reflection and reflective practice are an effective means of learning for the individual practitioner (Burnard, 1988; Coutts-Jarman, 1993 ) as well as a means of maintaining and improving the quality of care given in clinical practice ( Burnard, 1991). It was through the work of Argyris and Schon (1974) and latterly through Benner (1984) that reflection and reflective practice became fashionable within the education of nurses, midwives and health visitors.

## Reflection

There are many definitions in the literature of reflection, most however agree that it is an active, conscious process (Dewey, 1933; Boud, 1985; Schon, 1987 and Reid, 1993). Reflection is often initiated when the individual practitioner encounters some problematic aspect of practice and attempts to make sense of it.

Dewey (1933) defined reflection as:

*'An active persistent and careful consideration of any belief or supposed form of knowledge in the light of the*

*grounds that support it and the further conclusion to which it tends.'*

(Dewey, 1933: 9)

Dewey worked as an educationalist and developed his concept of reflective practice and reflection through *experiential learning* theories. He concluded in his work that the experience the individual lives through can be described as a dynamic continuum and that each experience influences the quality of future experiences.

Boud *et al* (1985) take a different perspective and define it as:

*'A generic term for those intellectual and effective activities in which individuals engage to explore their experiences in order to lead to a new understanding and appreciation.'*

(Boud *et al*, 1985: 19)

Boud and his co-writers view reflection from the learner's point of view. They emphasise the relationship of the reflective process and the learning experience against what the learner can do.

Schon (1987) in his work identifies two types of reflection, these are reflection-in-action — thinking on your feet, and reflection-on-action — retrospective thinking. He suggests that reflection is used by practitioners when they encounter situations that are unique, and when individuals may not be able to apply known theories or techniques previously learnt through formal education. Greenwood (1993), however, identifies weaknesses and inconsistencies in Argyris and Schon's work as they fail to follow their own recommendations. This, she argues, has resulted in the implementation and prescription of dubious strategies for the promotion of what Schon refers to as enlightened professional artistry. Often formal education cannot answer the complex questions of clinical practice and there remains a gap in knowledge gained. Schon, however, argues that wisdom can be learnt by reflection on dilemmas that are encountered in practice and that by using reflection-on-action practitioners can continue to develop their practice.

Reid (1993) in her definition also noted reflection as an active process rather than passive thinking. She states:

*'Reflection is a process of reviewing an experience of practice in order to describe, analyse, evaluate and so inform learning about practice.'*

(Reid, 1993: 305)

Kemmis (1985) agrees with Reid that the process of reflection is more than a process that focuses 'on the head'. It is, he argues, a positive active process that reviews, analyses and evaluates experiences, draws on theoretical concepts or previous learning and so provides an action plan for future experiences. Johns (1995) notes that reflection enables the practitioner to assess, understand and learn through their experiences. It is a personal process that usually results in some change for the individual in their perspective of a situation or creates new learning for the individual.

Reflection starts with the individual or group and their own experiences and can result, if applied to practice, in improvement of the clinical skills performed by the individual through new knowledge gained on reflection. Clamp (1980) noted that nurses' *attitudes* largely govern how care is administered to their client and the commonest causes of poor care are ignorance and inappropriate attitudes. This process of reflection, if then related into practice, can assist the individual in gaining the required knowledge, leading to a potential improvement in the *quality of the care* received from that individual. The outcome of reflection as identified by Mezirow (1981) is learning.

Louden (1991) describes in ordinary language reflection as:

*'Serious and sober thought at some distance from action and has connotations similar to "meditation" and "introspection". It is a mental process which takes place out of the stream of action, looking forward or (usually) back to actions that have taken place.'*

(Louden, 1991: 149)

# Reflective practice

Once we have decided what reflection is we can then look at reflective practice.

According to Reid (1993) reflective practice is:

*'Potentially both a way of learning and a mode of survival and development once formal education ceases.'*

(Reid, 1993: 307)

Jarvis (1992) refers to reflective practice as 'thoughtful practice', performing actions that are based on the known theory and monitoring consciously these actions, questioning why the outcomes occur and so identifying a widening legitimate knowledge base for the individual. Reflective practice can then not only assist in improving the quality of practice for the individual, but can also assist the individual practitioner in applying formal education and knowledge into clinical practice, thereby applying theory to practice and practice to theory. Reflective practice may also lead the practitioner into identifying and justifying their own theories and/or creating a new defensible knowledge.

Another aspect of reflective practice is that the individual can justify their practice through reflection on their experiences, being able to identify personal theories, values and beliefs and applying previous learnt knowledge to a given situation. Reflective practice when recorded can help to assist the individual in recognising and providing evidence of professional and personal development for use in their personal professional profiles.

# Learning through experience

Many pre registration and post registration nursing courses (ENB, 1989 and UKCC, 1986) have included reflective practice as an integral component of their programmes. They do not however identify how and when the process is to be incorporated.

If we are to use reflection in our experience we will need to readdress the issue of where knowledge comes from and how learning through experience is relevant to the practitioner.

Lewin (1951) in his work relating to social science identifies the complexity of factors that affect learning. He suggests that interaction affects the development of the individual's learning styles allowing them to know, explain and cope with the experiences they encounter.

Carper (1978) in her work identifies what she refers to as 'Patterns of Knowing'. She suggests four types:

1.  Scientific knowledge

2.  Personal knowledge

3.  Aesthetic knowledge

4.  Ethical knowledge.

It will be useful to review each of these ways of knowing individually as reflection and reflective practice will play a major role in gaining and providing evidence of learning through various learning experiences.

**Scientific knowledge**

This is what Schon (1983) refers to as 'technical rationality' and Burnard (1989) as 'factual knowledge'. This knowledge is gained in health care practice predominantly through formal education, reading and research. It is the science of nursing that can be taught through all courses at both pre and post registration levels. Scientific knowledge involves theories that can be learnt, they are involved with describing and predicting facts. This scientific knowledge is capable of replication and therefore given the scientific title.

**Personal knowledge**

This is the knowledge, acquired through life's experiences,

that the individual processes. Burnard (1989) refers to it as 'practice knowledge' and Benner (1984) discusses the acquisition of this knowledge through clinical practice. Personal knowledge can be used to identify the difference between what Benner refers to as 'the advanced beginner and the expert nurse'. This knowledge is often not scientifically based and can be generalised.

## Aesthetic knowledge

This is what Burnard (1989) refers to as 'experiential knowledge' and can be explained as the art of nursing. Benner (1984) in her work refers to the intuition gained through practice that the expert nurse learns through experience. Intuitive judgement is what distinguishes expert human judgement from the decisions or computations that might be made by a beginner or machine (Benner and Tanner, 1987). The aesthetic knowledge is gained through the analysis of the application of theory into practice. It is mainly through this type of knowledge that reflection and reflective practice can assist the individual practitioner in coming to terms with experiences and assist them in applying their scientific and personal knowledge into a given situation. The problems encountered with this area are that nursing has traditionally been based upon the scientific medical model. This sits uncomfortably with the idea of aesthetic knowledge. Reflective practice can challenge some of the teaching of health care and can fuel the art versus science debate of nursing practice.

## Ethical knowledge

This Benner refers to as the moral knowledge, gained through our lives, that we all hold. This knowledge is not to be confused with the legal or ethical knowledge learnt in formal training. These moral values may at times come into conflict with professional and legal requirements.

## Utilising reflection and reflective practice

Reflective practice can be used to identify, justify and assist with the appropriate application of theory to practice. This can assist the clinical practitioner in changing care given through a sound knowledge base presented to their client group. It may also provide the practitioner with written evidence of reflection for their personal and professional development in accordance with PREP. The written accounts may be used in the classroom to provide a means of applying theory into practice and to identify the application of the scientific and personal knowledge into practice. This may also be documented in a personal profile as evidence of learning through practice. The use of documented reflection and reflective practice will be discussed in the following chapters.

The Professional Code of Conduct (UKCC, 1992) for all nurses, midwives and health visitors identifies the need for individual practitioners to be able to justify their practice, and to know their limitations and construct their future action plans.

The Department of Health (NHSME, 1993) in their paper 'Vision for the Future' identifies the need to use reflective skills in their introduction of clinical supervision. With the introduction of clinical supervision, reflective practice is essential to identify areas of professional development and can be used as a forum to explore the relation of theory into practice. Gibbs (1988) states that reflection assists in the development of analytical skills moving practitioners away from the descriptive approach and therefore affecting how they perceive their practice. This process may then assist the individual in attaining the competence and supervisory skills required by the 'Vision for the Future' recommendations.

Reflective practice can also assist the individual in being able to identify for their own practice, the mismatch between the ideology of the profession and the reality of their clinical practice, giving them the ability to adapt and develop their practice in the real world.

Through reflection and reflective practice the individual utilises the ways of knowing, the scientific, personal, ethical and aesthetic knowledge drawing them together in order to facilitate the development of what Benner (1984) refers to as the 'expert practitioner' and the ENB (1995) identifies as the 'specialist practitioner'.

To conclude, Reid (1993) states that reflective practice is potentially a way of learning and a mode of survival and development for the individual after formal education has finished.

If nurses, health visitors and midwives are to gain knowledge across all the areas and to move their practice forward then reflective practice must play an active role in the development of that practice.

The development of reflection assists the individual to gain self awareness, insight, ability to express emotion and problem solving skills which are all desirable for professional growth according to Parker *et al* (1995).

# References

Argyris C, Schon D (1974) Theories of Action that Inhibit Individual Learning. *Amer Psychologist* **39**: 638–654

Benner P (1984) *From Novice to Expert*. Addison Wesley, California

Benner P, Tanner C (1987) How Expert Nurses use Intuition. *Amer J Nurs* **87** (1): 23–31

Boud D, Keough R, Walker D (1985) *Reflection: Turning Experience into Learning*. Kogan Page, London: 19

Burnard P (1988) The Journal as an assessment and Evaluation Tool in Nurse Education. *Nurse Ed Today* **8**: 105–107

Burnard P (1989) Developing Critical Ability in Nurse Education. *Nurse Ed Today* **9**: 271–275

Burnard P (1991) Improving Through Reflection. *J Dist Nurs* May: 10–11

Burnard P (1995) Nurse Educators Perceptions of Reflection and Reflective Practice. *J Adv Nurs* **21**: 1167–1174

Carper B (1978) Fundamental Patterns of Knowing. *Adv Nurs Sci* **1**: 13–23

Clamp C (1980) Learning Through Critical Incidents. *Nurs Times* Oct 2: 1755–1758

Coutts- Jarman J (1993) Using Reflection and Experience in Nurse Education. *BJN* **2** (1): 77–80

Dewey J (1933) *How we Think.* Henrey Regney, Chicago: 9

English National Board (1989) *Preparation of Teachers, Mentors and Supervisors to the context of Project 2000.* ENB, London

English National Board (1995) *Creating Lifelong Learners Partnerships for Care.* ENB, London

Ghaye A, Cuthbert S, Danai K, Dennis D (1996) *Learning through Critical Reflective Practice.* Pentaxion Ltd, Newcastle upon Tyne

Gibbs G (1988) *Learning by Doing: A guide to Teaching Learning Methods.* Oxford Polytechnical, Oxford

Greenwood J (1993) Reflective Practice: A Critique of the Work of Argyris and Schon. *J Adv Nurs* **21**: 1044–1050

Jarvis P (1992) Reflective Practice and Nursing. *Nurse Ed Today* **12** : 174–181

Johns C (1995) The Value of Reflective Practice for Nursing. *J Clinical Nurs* **4**: 23–30

Johns C (ed) (1994) *The Burford NDU Model: Caring in Practice.* Blackwell Science, London

Kemmis S (1985) Action Research and the Politics of Reflection. In: Boude D *et al* (1985) *Reflection Turning Experience into Learning.* Kogan Page, London

Lewin K (1951) *Field Theory in Social Science.* Harper Row, New York

Louden W (1991) *Understanding Teaching* . Cassell, London: 149

Mead G (1934) *Mind, Self and Society: From the Standpoint of Social Behaviourist.* Chicago Press

Mezirow J (1981) A Critical Theory of Adult Learning and Education. *Adult Education* **32** (1): 3–24

NHSME (1993) *A Vision for the Future — The Nursing, Midwifery and Health Visitors Contribution to Health Care.* Department of Health, London

Parker D, Webb J, D'Souza B (1995) The Value of Critical Incident Analysis as an Educational Tool and its Relationship to Experiential Learning. *Nurse Ed Today* **15**: 111–116

Reid B (1993) 'But we're Doing It Already!' Exploring a response to the concept of reflective practice in order to improve its facilitation. *Nurse Ed Today* **13**: 305–309

Schon D (1983) *The Reflective Practitioner: How Practitioners Think in Action*. Harper Collins, San Francisco

Schon D (1987) *Educating the Reflective Practitioner* . Josey Bass, San Francisco

UKCC (1986) *Project 2000: A New Preparation for Practice*. UKCC, London

UKCC (1990) *The Report of Post Registration Education and Practice Project*. UKCC, London

UKCC (1992) *Professional Code of Conduct*. UKCC, London

# 2
# A critique of models
# of reflection

If health care professionals view themselves or are viewed as 'technicians' and nursing as embracing Schon's notion of 'technical rationality', there would be little need for books on reflective practice. If, however, health care in general and nurses in particular see themselves as agents of progressive improvements in the quality of care, vision and compassion, the former position collapses and reflective practice becomes a genuinely compelling part of the transformative agenda. This chapter seeks to review a number of different models of reflection. By comparing one with another their similarities and differences will be highlighted. This process will combine a 'discourse of possibility' (what the models can offer us) with a 'discourse of critique' (the limitations of the models). This combination seeks to expose the power that models of reflection have to enable health care professionals to become more critically aware of their own values and the extent to which they live them out in their clinical practice. It also demonstrates the power models of reflection have to transform practice and the clinical context in which it is embedded.

## What are models of reflection?

We need to begin with a few broad brush strokes. Models of reflection are characterised by their number and variety. While some are explicitly called 'models of reflection' others are more generally called 'models of learning'. Additionally, some require the learner to engage in reflection on practice in a sustained and continuous manner while others include 'reflection' as part of a process which includes other actions or strategies such as gathering data about practice. Some models appear to place greater emphasis on explicating a 'process' of reflection while others imply that the process is a means to an end, that end being improvements in health care practice. Reflection can also concern itself with the micro aspects of our clinical work: a problematic client, improving a particular aspect of care, changing a routine and so on to more macro concerns about the culture of a hospital/Trust, ethical principles underlying practice, resource allocations and the like. Whether micro or macro in focus, reflection brings together issues of human agency and structure. In very general terms though, we could advance that models of reflection, no matter how they are constructed and what they require of us, do share the following qualities. They:

- Help us to learn from our experience because they are practitioner focused. As part of this process they help us to develop a greater sense of personal-professional biography and history.

- Engage us in the process of knowledge creation by helping us to move from tacit knowing to more conscious and explicit knowing.

- Help us to overcome professional inertia by asking us to look at what we do, our taken-for-granted clinical worlds and that which is atypical, 'critical' and professionally significant.

- Tend to add more meaning and ascribe new and relevant meaning to our clinical practice through reflective conversations with clinical situations. In this sense they enhance meaningful dialogue.

- Have some significance for future personal and sometimes collective future action.

- Celebrate the role of human agency.

We can summarise the commonalities between models of reflection by suggesting that all such models can be seen from one or more of the following perspectives.

*1. A competency-based perspective:* in that they are to do with clinical skill development, clinical action and improving practice within the contemporary world of the health care delivery system.

*2. A personal perspective:* in that they are to do with personal agendas, emotionality, self-study and individual enhancement through a greater sense of self worth and identity.

*3. An experiential perspective:* in that nurses are involved in an active exploration of experience, both their experience and that of others. This requires that they value their own experience and have an openness that enables them to learn from the experiences of others ( Kolb, 1984).

*4. A transformatory perspective:* in that they are to do with destabilisation because they challenge the status quo, challenge oppressive and disempowering clinical contexts and focus on reducing or removing barriers to improvement.

All the models reviewed in this chapter differentially and in particular ways address three overlapping and interacting worlds of the health care professional. They are the:

- **Social world**: For example ward, unit and department cultures or contexts to which reflection refers and in which reflection is located. This social world is made up of feelings, norms, attitudes and values.

- **Behavioural world**: For example routine and emergency work and the formal and informal rules and protocols which guide and give rise to competent clinical action.

- **Structural world**: For example the overarching internal and external politico-economic and socio-cultural power structures which govern and influence who gets what, where and how and which fundamentally determine the conditions under which health care professionals work.

These three worlds can be linked to Habermas's three generic learning domains (1971) namely the social, the technical and the emancipatory. These domains can be seen as broad ways of modelling reflective practice. The first can be related to personal meanings, to the artistry of generating interpersonal understanding and effective communication. The second to task-related competence, craft knowledge and to making more efficient what is already in existence. The third is more radical and has a political agenda in its desire to improve clinical practice through a transformation of current configurations of knowledge, social relations and values that give rise to particular patterns of practice.

One of the first questions that confront us is, 'which model of reflection should I use?' But let us be clear. There is no virtue in being a slave to any model. They should be viewed as catalysts for learning. Choice of a model is dependent upon criteria embedded in each of these conceptualisations*'of reflection'*.

## Some conceptualisations of reflection are;

- **As a dichotomy** of reflection-in-action and reflection-on-action (Schon, 1983, 1987). The latter is the concern of this text. Reflection-on-action is a retrospective interrogation of practice to come to know the knowledge used and the feelings that accompanied action within a particular clinical situation. The notion of 'reframing' lies at the heart of this conceptualsation. This is a process where data drawn from our practice is seen differently.

- **As intentional activity** (Ghaye, 1996a) in that we reflect on purpose and with a purpose in mind. It is no accident that we reflect. Something usually triggers it.

- **As knowledge and skill development** (Benner, 1984; Bloom, 1956; ENB, 1994; Gatley, 1992; Steinmaker and Bell, 1979) where reflection is claimed to develop and enhance particular cognitive, affective and psycho-motor skills.

- **As creating practitioner-derived knowledge** (Smyth, 1991) which is worthy, valid and relevant to particular clinical situations.

- **As resolving problematic situations** and the basis for problem-based learning (Dewey, 1933; Schon, 1991; Woods, 1994) where systematic reflection enables us to think through and resolve clinical situations which we perceive as being charcterised by uncertainty, disorder and indeterminacy.

- **As a process of becoming different** (Giroux, 1987) in which reflection helps us to equip ourselves with the lenses to read the world critically in order to improve it.

## Some purposes of reflection are;

- **To act as a bridge** (Silcock, 1994) from tacit knowledge to considered action and from the practice world to the process of theory generation.

- **To enhance the quality of action** (Olsen, 1992, Burrows, 1995) in that it enables us to talk about our clinical practice (critically reflective conversations with self and others) and to practice different things. Reflection without action is just 'wishful thinking' (Freire, 1972).

- **To increase accountability** (Diamond, 1991)
  because the principles of technocratic efficiency
  emphasise hierarchically structured, 'top down' models
  of acountability with an increasing burden for
  professional accountability residing with the individual
  health carer.

- **As a much needed counter-discourse** (Smyth,
  1991) to challenge the ensconced and pervasive
  technicist views of health care practice which
  marginalise and delegitimate the clinical experiences,
  histories and practical wisdom nurses use in mediating
  their lives.

## Categories of models of reflection

Our review of the literature on models of reflection has
enabled us to categorise them in five ways. All of them aim to
'guide' the reflective process but do so in different ways.
Some are more prescriptive, others give the nurse more
freedom to learn. The five models are:

- Structured
- Hierarchical
- Iterative
- Synthetic
- Holistic.

### Structured models

In Johns' work (1993, 1994a, 1994b) he explicitly talks about
reflection being a 'profoundly difficult thing to do without
expert guidance and support' (1994b). His intention in
constructing a model of guided reflection is to, 'enable
reflective practitioners to access, make sense of and to
subsequently learn through their experiences to become

more effective in their practices' (1994a). At the heart of his structured approach are questions. In fact, he describes the model as a series of cues. Figure 1 shows how the 'cue questions' fall into five groups and that they are of the 'what', 'why' and 'how' type. The model is structured in the sense that the questions are already prespecified and the health carer works through the set sequence of questions. Johns is insistent that because reflection on practice is often 'tough' and 'frustrating', that it 'should always be supervised or coached in order to support the journey' (1994b).

The central issues which arise from his model are those to do with the:

- Linearity of it and the tidy view of learning that this conveys

- Way questions are not owned by the health care professional but provided for them.

Smyth (1991) has developed another structured model characterised by what he calls 'a number of moments that can be linked to a series of questions' thus:

1. Describe:     what do I do?

2. Inform:      what does this description mean?

3. Confront:    how did I come to be like this?

4. Reconstruct: how might I do things differently?

## Figure 1.

The following cues are offered to help practitioners access, make sense of, and learn through experience

| | |
|---|---|
| **1** | **Description** |
| 1.1 | Write a description of the experience |
| 1.2 | What are the key issues within this description that I need to pay attention to? |
| **2** | **Reflection** |
| 2.1 | What was I trying to achieve? |
| 2.2 | Why did I act as I did? |
| 2.3 | What were the consequences of my actions: |
| | • for the patient and family? |
| | • for myself? |
| | • for the people I work with? |
| 2.4 | How did I feel about this experience when it was happening? |
| 2.5 | How did the patient feel about it? |
| 2.6 | How do I know how the patient felt about it? |
| **3** | **Influencing factors** |
| 3.1 | What internal factors influenced my decision making and actions? |
| 3.2 | What external factors infuenced my decision making and actions? |
| 3.3 | What sources of knowledge did or should have influenced my decision making and actions? |
| **4** | **Alternative strategies** |
| 4.1 | Could I have dealt better with the situation? |
| 4.2 | What other choices did I have? |
| 4.3 | What would be the consequences of these other choices? |
| **5** | **Learning** |
| 5.1 | How can I make sense of this experience in light of past experience and future practice? |
| 5.2 | How do I **now** feel about this experience? |
| 5.3 | Have I taken effective action to support myself and others as a result of this experience? |
| 5.4 | How has this experience changed my ways of knowing in practice? |
| | • empirics |
| | • ethics |
| | • personal |
| | • aesthetics |

Carper B (1978) Fundamental patterns of knowing in nursing. *Advances in Nursing Science* **1**: 13–23

Source: Johns C (1994a) Nuances of reflection in *Journal of Clinical Nursing* **3**: 71–75

The third moment is often the most problematic for it is here that practice has to be interrogated and questioned. It is where practice is given some legitimacy through a careful analysis of its genesis. As a way of providing more 'structure' to help in this confrontation process Smyth offers a 'series of guiding questions that might include the following':

- What do my practices say about my assumptions, values and beliefs?

- Where did these ideas come from?

- What social practices are expressed in these ideas?

- What is it which causes me to maintain my theories?

- What views of power do they embody?

- Whose interests seem to be served by my practices?

- What is it that acts to constrain my views of what is possible?

These questions get to the heart of the agency-structure debate. They are phrased in such a way that the forces that serve to liberate or constrain us in our practice are more known and not seen as immutable givens, but essentially contestable.

Whereas Johns' model is essentially about developing an epistemology of nursing practice, the work of Smyth and Habermas (1971) fuse epistemology with sociology and politics. Together they are concerned with the value-ladenness of practice, the interests certain practices serve and the structures of power that affect what we do in context. Basing his work on Freudian psychoanalysis and the power of reflection as a way of becoming more emancipated, Habermas proposes a model structured in 'four stages'.

| Stage 1 | A description and interpretation of the existing situation. |
|---|---|

Stage 2          A penetration of the reasons which
                 brought the existing situation to the
                 form that it takes.

Stage 3          An agenda for altering the situation.

Stage 4          An evaluation of the achievement of that
                 agenda in practice.

Some may argue that understanding a clinical situation
better is no guarantee that practice will indeed improve.
Similarly becoming more aware of the impediments to
improving practice does not lead us on naturally to
improving practice if we are powerless to act to remove these
impediments. It may be that the structured approaches of
Johns, Smyth and Habermas provide us with an optimistic
model. On the other hand are they overestimating the power
of reflection because of their lack of 'guidance' with regard to
becoming emancipated?

**Hierarchical models**

One of the best known models of this kind was developed by
Mezirow (1981) where reflection is presented in seven levels
with 'reflectivity' at the base of the hierarchy and
'theoretical' at the top (see Figure 2). As soon as reflection is
modelled in this way certain assumptions become apparent:
first that different types or kinds of reflection can indeed be
identified and described; second that one kind of reflection is
more complex than the preceding one; third that this
complexity is empirically verifiable; fourth that the benefits
from reflection accrue by climbing the 'ladder' or ascending
the hierarchy; fifth that 'mastery' at one level is a
prerequisite for moving onto the next level and finally that
learning develops by some process of inclusion in that later
levels encapsulate all that which has gone before.

**Figure 2.**

| Mezirow's Seven Levels of Reflection |
|---|
| **1.    Reflectivity** |
| The act of becoming aware of a specific perception, meaning or behaviour of your own or the habits you have of seeing, thinking and acting. |
| **2.    Affective** |
| Becoming aware of how you feel about the way you are perceiving, thinking or acting. |
| **3.    Discriminant** |
| Assessing the efficacy of your perceptions, thoughts and actions. Recognising the reality of the contexts in which you work and identifying your relationship to the situation. |
| **4.    Judgemental** |
| Making and becoming aware of your value judgements, about your perceptions, thoughts and actions, in terms of being positive or negative. |
| **5.    Conceptual** |
| Being conscious of your awareness and being critical of it (eg. being critical of the concepts you use to evaluate a situations). |
| **6.    Psychic** |
| Recognising in yourself the habit of making precipitant judgements about people based on limited information. |
| **7.    Theoretical** |
| Becoming aware of the influence of underlying assumptions upon your judgement. |

**(Mezirow, 1981)**

Models of this kind are a variant of a structured model with the underlying structural variable being based upon the notion of increasing complexity. Van Manen (1977) and Goodman (1984) have provided similar hierarchical models based upon three levels of reflection namely:

- Practices needed to reach given objectives
- Reflection of the links between principles and practice
- Reflection which incorporates the above and ethical and political concerns.

## Iterative models

These models are principally based upon the idea that the reflective process is most appropriately described as a 'cycle' and that deepening awareness, increases in knowledge and skilfulness arise from repeated 'clockwise' movements around the reflective cycle. Gibbs (1988) provides a general cyclical model having six stopping points with each point on the cycle being associated with a key question (see Figure 3).

**Figure 3**

**Description**
What happened?

**Feelings**
What were you
thinking and feeling?

**Action plan**
If it arose again
what would you do?

**Reflective Cycle**

**Evaluation**
What was good and bad
about the experience?

**Conclusion**
What else could
you have done?

**Analysis**
What sense can you make of
the situation?

**(Gibbs, 1988)**

In iterative models the ongoing nature of learning begins to aappear Unlike the previous two model types, reflective cycles have an 'unfinished business' feel to them. Out of the stopping point called 'action plan' comes new clinical actions, encounters and situations that can be understood by again asking the question 'what happened?'

Atkins and Murphy ( 1994) draw upon the work of others to develop their own cyclical model (see Figure 4). Although they state that it is possible to begin the reflective process by reflecting on achievements, their model is drawn so that it explicitly shows the process starting with an 'awareness of uncomfortable feelings and thoughts'. To the inexperienced

**Figure 4.**

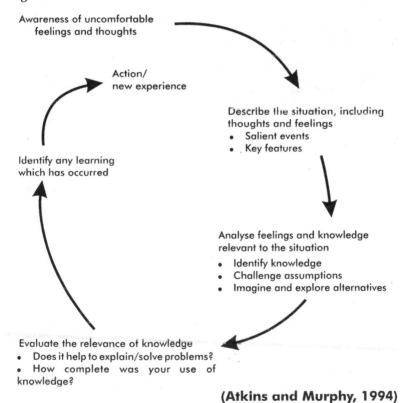

Awareness of uncomfortable
feelings and thoughts

Action/
new experience

Describe the situation, including
thoughts and feelings
- Salient events
- Key features

Identify any learning
which has occurred

Analyse feelings and knowledge
relevant to the situation
- Identify knowledge
- Challenge assumptions
- Imagine and explore alternatives

Evaluate the relevance of knowledge
- Does it help to explain/solve problems?
- How complete was your use of knowledge?

**(Atkins and Murphy, 1994)**

eye their cyclical model conveys the message that reflection always starts with something 'negative', 'uncertain' and 'unsatisfactory'. Its strength, like Gibbs (1988), lies in the fact that it endeavours to incorporate knowledge, feelings and action in one learning cycle.

**Figure 5.**

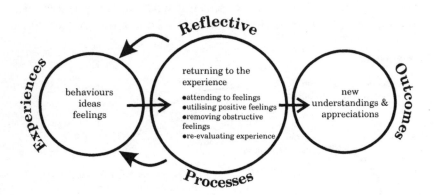

**(Boud *et al*, 1985)**

There are two main variants on the basic iterative model. The first by Boud *et al* (1985) captures, among other things, more of the messiness of learning through reflection (see Figure 5). Their model cleverly holds one cycle, of three parts, together with two movements. First there is a cycle which essentially moves anti-clockwise. Here the learner revisits earlier experiences. Then there is another process which moves forward and connotes that reflection is not just a retrospective process but also a prospective one. The central cycle is characterised by the processes of deconstruction and reconstruction. The second variant is captured in the action research literature (Ghaye *et al*, 1996b) (see Figure 6). This is worth mentioning for three reasons. First because the notion of a cycle of learning is made more complex and presented as a 'learning spiral'.

**Figure 6.**

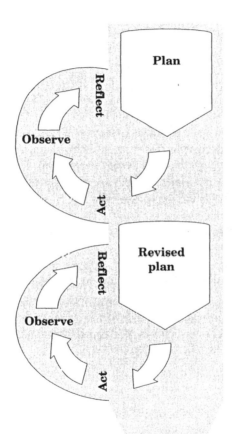

**(Ghaye *et al*, 1996b)**

The second is that reflection is just one 'moment' in the spiral process. The moments are:

- Plan
- Act
- Observe
- Reflect
- Replan.

The third is that the spiral conveys a clear message that having gone through these moments we never return to the same place and start again. The planning, acting, observing and reflecting at least move our thinking forward if not our clinical practice or the context in which it is located.The problem is that we need to be able to validate any claims we make that indeed we have moved on.

**Synthetic models**

In an excellent text by Louden (1991) we find a very useful synthetic model of reflection. By synthetic we mean that in attempting 'to clear a conceptual path through the variety of ways in which the term reflection has been employed' he has brought together, in one holistic model, two of the critical aspects of reflection, namely:

- The **interests** of reflection: these are the goals or ends of the act of reflection.
- The **forms** of reflection: these are the characteristics of the act of reflection.

In Figure 7 we see that this synthetic model builds on Habermas's (1971) framework and is portrayed as a four-by-four matrix. The two dimensions of the matrix, he argues, are both different and complementary. What is important to grasp is that each act of reflection has both an interest and a form. Louden identifies four types in 'interest' which we have applied to health care. These are:

**Technical:**   an interest in standards, competencies and the development of technical skills.

**Personal:**   an interest in personal meaning and understanding and how this shapes how we feel and act.

**Problematic:**   an interest in the resolution of problems of clinical action.

**Critical:**   an interest in questioning taken-for-granted thoughts, feelings and actions.

**Figure 7.**

**Forms**

| | Introspection | Replay and rehearsal | Enquiry | Spontaneity |
|---|---|---|---|---|
| Technical | | | | |
| Personal | | | | |
| Problematic | | | | |
| Critical | | | | |

**Interests**

**(Louden, 1991)**

The four 'forms' of reflection are:

*Introspection*: which is similar to Schon's reflection-on-action in that it is deliberate contemplation of a past event at some distance from the stream of action.

*Replay and Rehearsal*: where events are reworked in our heads, gone over again and might also involve the nurse talking about an event that has happened or which might happen in the future.

*Enquiry*: where there is a deliberate and explicit connection between thinking and doing. This lies close to a tenet of action research in that it is a planned intervention, a deliberate move to systematically look into something.

*Spontaneity*: where reflection is so bound up in the moment of the action that there is no conscious awareness of thinking about the action. It is tacit reflection which takes place within the stream of experience. It is what Schon would call reflection-in-action.

One of the strengths of this model is that it helps us to appreciate what other models do and can offer us. For example we can now review the previous three model types and interrogate them with questions of the kind, 'do they connect a single interest with a single form?', 'do they connect a single interest with a range of forms?' and so on. This model also acts as a catalyst in that it invites us to think about how separate and exhaustive the boxes and categories are. Finally the synthetic model allows us to appreciate some of the subtleties of learning from experience as in the course of one conversation with a mentor, clinical supervisor or preceptor, a nurse may move from a focus on one form and interest to another.

## An holistic model

As with synthetic models, holistic models which are flexible and explicitly values-based have yet to become established in the reflective development of health care professionals. Figure 8 is an example of a holistic model. Here Ghaye (1996a) argues that a model of reflective practice should align itself with a complex and dynamic  health care system and a rapidly changing health care environment. In a range of texts Ghaye *et al*, (1996c) set out what they call their model of the 'practitioner-as-learner' where reflection facilitates improvements in the quality of an individual's work and they link this closely with improvements in practice areas themselves. The model is an 'opportunity to learn' and is premised upon the idea that learning is enhanced through critical reflection and further, that critical reflective practice does make a difference. Their holistic model embraces eight learning principles. These are that:

* The model is enabling rather than prescriptive.

* Reflection should begin with a consideration of individual and collective professional values and what it means to be a professional and that after this the learner is free to engage in any other reflective cycle as long as the choice is a conscious and justifiable one.

* Improving practice requires the health care professional to see holistically and think in a multidisciplinary way.

* Improving practice requires a high level of skill in being able to transfer, apply and customise knowledge from other fields.

* Just as work conditions change so do the concepts and categories that we use to make sense of our professional practice. This requires nurses to interrogate the ways in which they habitually make

sense of their practice.

- Reflective and reflexive practice must interact if meaningful, relevant and sustainable improvement is to take place.
- Improving practice requires us to reflect upon the very nature or essence of our professionalism.

- Practice can be improved and learning facilitated through the establishment and nourishment of a community of reflective health care professionals engaging in peer group dialogue.

**Figure 8.**

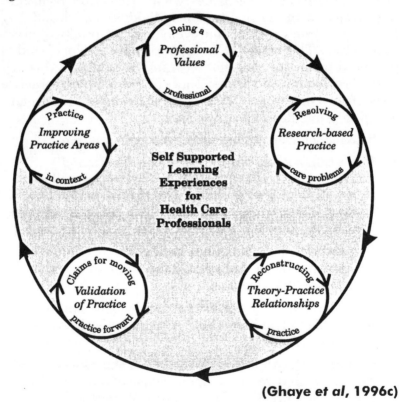

**(Ghaye et al, 1996c)**

For Ghaye *et al* (1996a) critically reflective practice involves questioning:

- Accepted understanding about health care practice
- Received 'truths' about the nature and power of individual and collective competence
- The relevance and generation of 'know-that', 'know-how' and 'know-why' knowledge.

Reflection is a complex business. This holistic model captures this complexity and gives the health carer the freedom to learn within an enabling framework, places the responsibility for learning on the shoulders of the individual or group of learners and also explicitly addresses the ethical dimension of reflecting on practice. Individuals are encouraged to monitor improvements in their thinking and clinical practice by periodically checking where they 'feel they are at' on a five-by-five matrix (see Figure 9). The vertical axis shows five different types of 'reflection-on-practice'. The horizontal axis shows five reflective cycles which together comprise this holistic model. They are cycles which focus learning on:

- 'My professional values'
- 'Researching my practice and resolving care problems'
- 'Looking at my practice in relation to the work of others'
- 'Setting out and supporting a claim that my practice has moved forward'
- 'Trying to improve my practice area'.

| Figure 9. Types of reflection | Cycle 1 Professional Values: being a professional | Cycle 2 Research-Based Practice: resolving care problems | Cycle 3 Theory-Practice Relationships: reconstructing practice | Cycle 4 Validation of Practice: claims for moving practice forward | Cycle 5 Improving Practice Areas: practice in context |
|---|---|---|---|---|---|
| **Critical** | Able to evaluate the link between own professional development and organisational improvement. Can question organisational practice and policy constructively but critically, to reveal contradictions between organisational rhetoric and realities. Can construct rationale for transforming organisational culture to make it more emancipatory and empowering. | Reflect fully upon the moral and ethical implications of research-based practice. Draws upon research to enlighten, empower and challenge their own and others' practice. Uses research to point to individual and collective contradictions in practice. Reflects upon the way research can constructively challenge the status quo. | Sees theory as able to question clinical habits, traditions and prevailing ideologies. Uses theory to enlighten their practice and emancipate it from the causal influences and structures that constrain it. Clearly able to 'theorise' about those things that constrain or liberate their practice. | Able to evaluate personal and collective claims for moving practice forward by linking them to notions of enlightenment, emancipation and empowerment. Can critique claims by adopting a position of reflective scepticism and by using both dialogical and dialectical thinking. | Able to synthesise individual and collective improvements with systemic and cultural improvements in the organisation. Can evaluate links between enhanced professionalism, improvements in practice, and more empowered health carers. Can conceptualise and critique workplace improvement as a democratic struggle about rights, fairness, justice and improved care. |
| **Interactive** | Able to link contradictions in practice to action plans for individual and collective improvement. Thorough understanding of internal/external influences that impact on own professional values and practice area values. Can articulate political and ethical consequences of action plans to improve thinking and practice. | Able to articulate the reasons why research-based practice is important. Through reflection, can link research with improvements in health care in their own practice area. Able to plan, implement and evaluate collaborative practice-based research. Opens up research so that others may critique it. Appreciates how value-laden the research process is. Uses the outcomes of research to reflect upon the nature of the relationship between practice and theory. | Able to articulate an interactive view of the relationship between theory and practice. Can justify a position that practice is theory-laden. Able to generate and defend their own practical theory. | Can set up validation events. Able to link the construction of a claim with the process of validating claims by self and through a peer group validation event. Can act in the role of critical friend. Can initiate, sustain and evaluate the critical dialogues that arise through the validation process. | Able to articulate links between desired improvements in the quality of action and improvements in client care. The impact of the improvement effort on all concerned can be justified. Thorough understanding of the influences on 'total quality'. Able to develop, implement and evaluate action plans to improve practice area culture. |

| | | | | | |
|---|---|---|---|---|---|
| **Receptive** | Can publicly justify practice with reference to personal and organisational values. Can identify self as a living contradiction and present evidence to illuminate this. Able to position personal values in relation to personal history, others' practice and the professional literature. Able to critique own espoused values and values-in-action. | Can justify what to research and how to do it. Through reflection, can identify and explain the problem, issue, concern or question they wish to research. Able to position their 'new' knowledge relative to other relevant research. Appreciates the importance of research being systematic, rigorous and valid. | Is able to justify where their own health care knowledge comes from. Can make sound connections between 'know how to', and 'know why' knowledge. Able to make judgements about the knowledge they and others should possess. Does not 'position' theory as opposite to practice, but integrated with practice. Able to articulate and explain links between 'what they say' and 'what they do'. | Able to publicly justify, in a clearly understandable manner, a claim that personal thinking and/or practice has moved forward. Able to distinguish between particular and general claims. Can position own claim in relation to other claims found in the professional literature. Able to make a reasoned judgement about the validity of others' claims. | Can publicly justify improvements to personal practice. Distinguishes between change and improvement and can present evidence to illuminate this. Sees improvement as a complex political and moral enterprise. Able to position personal improvement efforts in relation to literature on organisational development and training. |
| **Perceptive** | Developing consciousness of the significance and nature of professional values that give practice a shape, form and purpose. Can link descriptions of practice with explanations of practice, but not tie these into personal value positions. Personal practice events explained in relation to past practice and personal feelings towards practice. | Feels that research is intimidating, rather abstract, and often does not help them to resolve 'everyday' practice-based problems. Feels that it is the responsibility of others to generate/extend the knowledge base of the profession. Feels poorly equipped to undertake 'serious' research. Feels under pressure to make their practice more accountable and evidence-based. Feels research is for others, whilst practice is for them. | Enjoys the world of practice and is intimidated by theory. Feels that theory is abstract and practice is more concrete. Feels under pressure to use theory to justify their practice. Believes that a gap between theory and practice is right and natural. Feels that theory is acquired out of the workplace and has to be 'fitted' to practice. Does not feel equipped to defend a view that their practice is theory-laden. | Knows which areas of practice they feel (un)comfortable with, and can explain this. Aware of the significance and value-ladenness of the phrases 'making a claim' and 'validating practice'. Can express personal feelings about moving practice forward and the effects of routine, busyness, availability of professional development opportunities, family commitments etc on their practice. | Can articulate those aspects of personal practice which provoke anxiety, joy and so on. Can explain improvements with reference to personal experience. Knows that some get hurt in the improvement process. Improvement seen principally as a social business involving people and their feelings. Also improvement as 'doing the right thing', thus involving values, choices and dilemmas. |
| **Descriptive** | Tacit awareness of practice guided by professional values. Can describe practice — the 'what' and 'how' — accurately and comprehensively. Can contextualise practice. Able to present a vivid portrayal of self as a professional. | Can describe health care problems and can give a personal view about their resolution. Does not research their own practice. Mainly reads research papers when attending continuing education courses. Often caricatures research as 'grand', 'high status', involving large samples' and 'hypotheses'. Thinks research is something done by others. Has a tacit awareness of the importance of research for enhancing good practice. | Can give a personally meaningful definition of the term 'practical knowledge' and can relate this to concrete examples drawn from clinical practice. Describes practice mainly in terms of common-sense ways of knowing. Sees knowledge as 'outsider'. Knowledge is applied to practice. Can describe how knowledge has been acquired in training. Separates practice and theory. | Can describe what is known and how worthy they claim this knowledge is. Has a tacit awareness of the multiple meanings of 'practice', and the different ways that knowledge of and for practice is generated. Able to describe own practice and identify areas where practice has moved forward over time. Descriptions tied closely with professional biography and clinical interests. | Awareness that improvements in personal practice can be made. Tacit acknowledgement of the complexity of the improvement process. Can describe personally desirable improvements and contextualise them. Improvement seen principally as doing it right, as more of the same, just better. Improvement is seen mainly as a technical business. |

(Ghaye et al, 1996c)

In judging the worthwhileness and usefulness of each of these models the following should be borne in mind. Some models of reflection appear to be value-neutral or value-blind in that they do not talk about professional values. Some models focus on practice deficits and tend to convey a message that they need only to be used when something goes wrong. Some models present learning through reflection as a tidy, one-way and unproblematic process. What are the strictures in the structures, hiccups in the hierarchies and calamities in the cycles? Some appear to be trapped in a psychologistic framework ignoring health care as a moral and ethical art form, while others focus only on the private, individual and particular clinical world, not the wider public world of social and political action. Some emphasise self-understanding which may not be a basis for altering the existing structures and arrangements. Some emphasise personal deliberation and contemplation rather than active, militant confrontations with practice infused with understandings of power and politics. Finally, some models of reflection place a greater emphasis on self empowerment while others are more focused on critique and possibility. Above all else each model has strengths and limitations.

In some ways each of these five types of model of reflection can claim that they have the potential to:

- Foster the development of a more emancipated, enlightened and empowered health care professional

- Develop certain individual virtues like justice, honesty and courage

- Cast the health carer in the active role of meaning-maker

- Resolve contradictions and conflicts in clinical practice

- Link issues of human agency with structure.

However the continued use of models of reflection will only

occur if we are able to present valid claims that learning through reflection improves the quality of client care. Much more research needs to be done to support such a claim.

# References

Atkins S, Murphy K (1994) Reflective Practice. *Nurs Standard* **8** (39): 49–56

Benner P (1984) *From Novice to Expert*. Addison Wesley, New York

Bloom B (1956) *A Taxonomy of Educational Objectives*. McKay, New York

Boud D *et al*(1985) Promoting Reflection in Learning: A Model. In: Boud D, Keogh R, WalkerD (Eds) *Reflection: Turning Experience into Learning*. Kogan Page, New York

Burrows D (1995) The nurse teacher's role in the promotion of reflective practice. *Nurs Ed Today* **15**: 346–50

Dewey J (1933) *How we think: a Restatement of the Relation of Reflective Thinking to the Educative Process*. Heath & Co. New York

Diamond P (1991) *Teacher Education as Transformation*. Open University Press, Milton Keynes.

English National Board (1994) *Creating Lifelong Learners: Partnerships for Care*. ENB, London

Freire P (1972) *Pedagogy of the Oppressed*. Penguin, Harmondsworth

Gatley E (1992) PREPP: From Novice to Expert. *BJN* **1** (2): 88–91

Ghaye T (1996a) *An Introduction to Learning through Critical Reflective Practice*. Pentaxion Ltd, Newcastle upon Tyne

Ghaye T *et al*(1996b) *Research-based Practice: Resolving Care Problems*. Pentaxion Ltd, Newcastle upon Tyne

Ghaye T *et al*(1996c) *Learning through Critical Reflective Practice: Self-supported Learning Experiences for Health Care Professionals*. Pentaxion Ltd, Newcastle upon Tyne

Gibbs G (1988) *Learning by Doing: A guide to teaching and learning methods*. Further Education Unit, Oxford Brookes University, Oxford

Giroux H (1987) Educational Reform and the Politics of Teacher Empowerment. *New Ed* **9** (1–2): 3–13

Goodman J (1984) Reflection in Teacher Education: A case study and theoretical analysis. *Interchange* **15** (3): 9–26

Habermas J (1971) *Knowledge and Human Interests*. Heinemann, London.

Johns C (1993) Professional Supervision. *J Nurs Manag* **1**: 9–18

Johns C (1994a) Nuances of Reflection. *J Clinical Nurs* **3**: 71–75

Johns C (1994b) Guided Reflection. In: Palmer A, Burns S, Bulman C (Eds) (1994). *Reflective Practice in Nursing: The Growth of the Professional Practitioner*. Blackwell Scientific Publications, Oxford

Kolb D (1984) *Experiential Learning: Experience as the Source of Learning and Development*. Prentice Hall, New Jersey

Louden W (1991) *Understanding Teaching*. Cassell, UK

Mezirow J (1981) A critical theory of adult learning and education. *Adult Ed* **32** (1): 3–24

Olsen J (1992) *Understanding Teaching*. Open University Press, Milton Keynes

Schon D (1983) *The Reflective Practitioner: how professionals think in action*. Temple Smith, London.

Schon D (1987) *Educating the Reflective Practitioner*. Jossey-Bass, San Francisco

Schon D (ed) (1991) *The Reflective Turn: Case Studies in and on Educational Practice*. Teachers College Press, New York

Silcock P (1994) The Process of Reflective Teaching. *Brit J Ed Stud* **42** (3): 273–85

Smyth J (1991) Teachers as Collaborative Learners. Open University Press, Milton Keynes

Steinmaker N, Bell N (1979) *The Experiential Taxonomy — A new approach to teaching and learning*. Academic Press, London.

Van Manen M (1977) Linking ways of knowing with ways of being practical. *Curriculum Enquiry* **6** (3): 205–28

Woods D (1994) *Problem-based Learning: How to gain the most from PBL*. McMaster University Press, Hamilton, Ontario

# Section B

# Processes

# 3

# Enhancing learning through journal writing

The term a 'journal' often means different things to different people. (Holly, 1987, 1989; Ballantyne and Packer, 1995). It is more commonly associated with references to 'diaries', 'learning logs' and 'experiential workbooks'. It is dangerous to use these terms synonymously for there are shades of difference between them. Although they can all claim to enhance learning, each one can also claim to place a different emphasis on the role of self and others in the learning process, on how private or public the document is, on the formality or informality of it, the structure of each entry, how learning emerges and who might benefit. This chapter sets out our conception of a learning journal for health care professionals. The discussion focuses upon responses to a series of questions we are most frequently asked about learning through journal writing.

## Why should I keep a Professional Learning Journal?

There are political, professional and personal reasons for keeping a learning journal. Politically there is much being written about improvements in the health of the nation (DoH,1989a,1989b,1993). Embedded in these policy statements are rallying cries for each registered nurse, midwife and health visitor to be personally accountable for their practice. Keeping a learning journal is a way of developing the skills to become more accountable. The journal can be a repository for professional experiences which can be interrogated, deconstructed and re-evaluated to deepen awareness, enrich skilfulness and enable the health carer to construct robust justifications for their practice and valid arguments for improving their practice areas.

There are three very important professional reasons for keeping a learning journal. The first is the belief that journal writing is a **necessary skill for lifelong learning**. Recently the ENB has given increasing emphasis to education as a lifelong learning process (ENB 1991, 1994). Enmeshed in this discourse are descriptions of lifelong learners as 'change agents' and 'creative' practitioners who are 'responsible and accountable' for their work. The learning that can arise from keeping a journal has the potential to develop these qualities. The notion of a learning journal is now firmly embedded in the practice of nurse education. In essence it helps the health carer to develop the ability to be realistic judges of their own performance and through the writing process, to monitor what they claim to know and what remains to be known and practised.

The second reason is that journal writing is **necessary for effective clinical learning**. Effective learning:

*'involves learners being able to influence their own learning rather than waiting for others to do so, that is, being proactive. Those who are dependent on the continued impetus of teachers or workplace supervisors to develop and assess their knowledge and skills are severely handicapped in their learning.'*

(Boud, 1996: 14–15)

This second reason has huge implications for the individual

health carer, those responsible for the management of pre and post registration courses and for those involved in clinical supervision, mentoring and preceptorship. This second reason raises issues about promoting and acquiring learning-how-to-learn skills, about autonomy and self-direction, about responsibilities for learning and about the role of critical reflection in the interrogation and reconstruction of practice.

The third reason is that journal writing has the potential to **add value to pre and post registration courses**. The added value arises principally from the way the journal helps the nurse to focus attention on the impact the course has on them. In this way the journal has something important to contribute to the professionalisation of the health carer, the development of status and confidence. It adds value because it can act as a bridge between the knowledge, skills and sensitivities the nurse is acquiring on the one hand and their application and impact in the clinical environment on the other.

There are a host of personal reasons why it is currently opportune to keep a learning journal. If enhancing practice is about personal improvement linked to organisational development and meaningful, conscious action, then the art of critical reflection becomes a pre-requisite. Reflection touches a need within the professional to make sense of their situation. Keeping a learning journal is a way tacit knowledge can be set out for inspection and interrogation. It is a way of turning experience into learning.

Learning through journal writing illustrates our understanding of both the nature and generation of health care knowledge. In promoting learning journals we are advocating the view that reality is a social construction. (Berger and Luckmann, 1976; Guba and Lincoln, 1989). By this we are suggesting three things. First, that to act in a responsible, ethical and competent manner we need to understand and practice with good intentions in our clinical worlds. To do this we need to be aware that each of us, regardless of whether we work in the same area of clinical specialism, apprehends the world differently. So reality is not a fixed and universally agreed, objective reality. Reality differs from individual to individual and these differences arise because of our differing expectations, experience, intentions, values and so on. Secondly, we believe that we all exist in a social world. Our clinical action occurs in social spaces which are a web of human relationships comprised of such things as traditions, norms, roles, protocols, power relationships, class and gendered space. Thirdly, competent practice suggests that we try to apprehend the reality of our everyday clinical worlds as an ordered reality. In doing so we build or construct a world which has personal meaning and in which we can act competently and responsibly. Reality is not simply 'there', neutral and self-evident to all, but has to be apprehended and personally constructed. The process of journal writing is one of reality construction.

Our practice often occurs in a turbulent, changing and chaotic environment, in organisations where oppressive politico-social structures often constrain our working lives. Critical reflective practice, enhanced through journal writing, and with its prime concerns of a more enlightened, emancipated and empowered professional, helps us to recognise the structures that constrain and those which enable and facilitate. Through journal writing we can come to know what can be influenced and improved and in what ways.

The learning journal can be 'positioned' in the growing field of narrative research and is a way of understanding how individuals and groups of health care professionals experience and live out their professional lives. The learning journal helps us to define and redefine our purposes, locate and reconstruct our values and to fix our affective orientation to people and things within our organisation. In this sense the learning journal is concerned with developing an epistemology of health care practice. It focuses on learning from experience and on making sense of the practical events in our professional lives. It enables us not only to describe and explain our practice but also to justify it.

Knowledge generated through keeping a journal is also about the problematic areas of truth-seeking, the professional as researcher in their own clinical context and about action as a technical and moral enterprise.

## What do I put into a Learning Journal?

A learning journal should contain practical knowledge (Ghaye *et al*, 1996a) and wisdom and needs to be understood in content and process terms. *What* is written about, the phenomenon in other words, is the content. When written down a 'text' is created which enables nurses to re-examine fundamental issues associated with their professional identity and the contexts which mould it. The text can utilise historical, emotional, personal and clinical data in a creative and interpretative manner so that the meanings, which reveal themselves from the re-examination of journal entries at a later date, can inform current and future clinical practice.

*How* the phenomenon is written about, the mediums and genres used, is the writing process. Learning accrues from this process and is facilitated by responses to questions such as, 'what kind of health care professional am I?', 'how have I come to practice in this way?' and 'how can I improve my practice?' McNiff reflects on how writing can help to make learning happen:

> *'In writing I tap my tacit knowledge.... My writing becomes both symbolic expression of thought (this is what I mean) and the critical reflection on that thought (do I really mean this?) My writing is both reflection on action (what I have written) and reflection in action (what I am writing). The very act of making external, through the process of writing, what is internal,.... allows me to formulate explicit theories about the practices I engage in intuitively.'*
>
> (McNiff, 1990: 56)

Health care professionals know their practical worlds in general, social and shared ways and also in unique and personal ways. In constructing accounts of practice the past is not irrelevant but provides a context for present thinking and action and future intentions. The practical knowledge that characterises the content of a learning journal reaffirms the view that health carers hold and actively use knowledge of this kind to guide their clinical action and shape their practice area. Entries in the learning journal, if done systematically over time, provide an opportunity to appreciate more richly that this practical knowledge is something which is dynamic, held in an active relationship with practice and is something which gives it its shape, form and purpose.

You can write about 'critical learning incidents'. These are events or situations which are professionally significant to you. They may, on further reflection, mark a significant change or turning point in your learning. They may cause you to stop and think about what you believe in, say and do. (see chapter 6). You can write about your 'educational/professional values'. Values make you the kind of professional that you are (Ghaye *et al*, 1996b). They provide a rationale for what you do. You can write about how far you are able to live out your values in your work, what helps and hinders this. You can write about the contradictions between what you say and do.

Learning journals serve many purposes which in turn conditions what you write in them. For example they can serve as a data collection tool for examining changes in your self-image, as an evaluation mechanism for aspects of your practice, to facilitate critical thinking, to release feelings and frustrations, to see different 'truths' and to develop observational skills. Above all else the learning journal should contain what is most relevant and meaningful to you and should do so in a form that you find most liberating. You do not have to write an essay for every entry! It can be jottings, annotated drawings with some writing underneath, concept maps, and so on. You need to set out your entry in sufficient detail that enables you to look back into it and understand things, as they were, at a later date. You might write in a file or a notebook. It is often useful to work out how you could add new thoughts and perspectives to earlier entries. For example you might write on the opposite side or reverse side of the paper in your file or add new pages to it to make it an ever expanding learning journal! It is important to give each entry a date and time.

In the work of Thomas (1992) we can find a number of issues and arguments which can be applied to the nature and educative potency of learning through journal writing. We have drawn upon his work and our own to develop a number of 'portraits' of 'The Clinical/Professional Learning Journal'.

### Portrait 1: The learning journal as 'A collection of anecdotes'

Personal anecdotes are experiences and so have a value. A collection of anecdotal evidence may reveal something worthwhile about clinical thinking, feelings and practice. To be more useful the anecdotes need to be placed in a context and need to be re-visited, re-read and evaluated over time. If anecdotes tell you nothing about how to improve what you do, then you need to change the content and process.

### Portrait 2: The learning journal as 'An interpreted story'

Just as stories have structures, entries in a journal can be structured also. An entry must have a clear beginning and a middle. It might not have an end, just more 'chapters'. As with story-making the content needs to be carefully selected and certain aspects of the entry given more emphasis than others. Storying also implies telling and listening which in turn relates to the ethical issue of consent (see below). Finally, journal entries of this kind, just like stories, have to be interpreted. Out of this comes the learning.

## Portrait 3: The learning journal as 'A fulcrum for professional development'

Some of the characteristics of learning-enriched clinical environments are collegiality, open communication, trust, support and help. Having the time to talk through the problems of practice is also a vital ingredient of both personal and collective professional development. For some the learning journal fulfils a need to tell, to enter into dialogues and to expose and explore various interpretations of 'this is what I did, for these reasons. This is what it felt like, so what do you think?'.

## Portrait 4: The learning journal as 'A means of asserting that your practice is evidence based'

This can be done if entries are guided by the following:

(a) That you are trying to live out the things you believe in

(b) That you wish to account for your actions

(c) That you are actively seeking to improve your practice

(d) That you acknowledge that claims for moving practice forward have to be supported with evidence.

## Portrait 5: The learning journal as 'A means of bringing order to turbulent clinical environments'

Practice areas have been described as being busy, dis/empowering, un/predictable, confusing, stressful, routine and unique. In trying to make sense of our practice worlds we need to hold the turbulence still for a moment. A single journal entry is a piece of frozen text waiting to be reflected upon. For a moment it brings a kind of order to things. Health care professionals are not confronted with

issues, challenges, dilemmas and problems that are in-
dependent of each other, but with dynamic, turbulent and
often chaotic situations which interact simultaneously.
Ackoff (1979) calls such situations 'messes'. Journal writing
has the potential to deepen our understanding of such
'messes'.

### Portrait 6:  The learning journal as 'A means of searching for the truth'

Each journal entry should not be viewed as some absolute,
fixed and verifiable truth, the last and final word on the
clinical matter under consideration. In our value-laden
practice worlds truths are often partial, contested, inter-
subjective and illusive. It is through the journal writing
process that we can come to appreciate our own perhaps
altering views and the opinions others hold about the same
clinical phenomenon.

### Portrait 7:  The learning journal as 'A basis for building a better world'

Journals should have a prospective quality. Constructive and
critical reflections on past events should constitute a new
beginning or an action plan to improve what is already being
experienced and in existence. Journal writing interpreted in
this way is situated in the realm of the good.

## When do I write my learning journal?

You should  aim to write regularly and at least once each
week. Learning has to be given a chance to emerge so you
need to make a series of entries and then re-read them to
search for patterns, themes, issues, conflicts and so on. It is
often useful to keep a small notebook to jot down the essence
of interesting, satisfying, worrying and/or puzzling encounters and conversations as you go through the week. You
can then elaborate upon them in your learning journal later.

## What are the ethical implications of keeping a learning journal?

If health care is about helping clients with ethically-laden health issues and decisions and if we caricature it as being interlaced with ethical dilemmas arising from practice (Bowman, 1994) then it is not surprising that enhancing learning through journal writing implies not only cognitive activity but also the need to embrace the process as a moral and ethical enterprise. Moving thinking and clinical practice forward requires not only expertise and commitment but also honesty and integrity. Put in its simplest form ethics is about issues of right and wrong and good and bad. (Burnard and Morrison, 1994; Burnard and Chapman, 1993). But ethics is a complex field and in the context of learning journals we are lured into considerations of rationality, reason, 'right action', fairness, justice, equality, reciprocity and rules. We have grouped the ethical issues associated with journal writing under three headings. These are rights, risks and benefits, and consent.

### The issue of rights

If you reflect on your practice through your learning journal you have certain rights. These relate to ideas of self-respect, self-esteem and dignity. Whether or not you keep your journal entries to yourself or share them in some way, you have the right to self-determination. You should not be coerced into making public what is written in your journal. You have the right to privacy. You should be the one who determines the time, extent and context under which you disclose your journal entries. You have the right to decide what you withhold and what you share. You also have the right to assume that the content of the entries you make public will be kept confidential. If you share the contents of your journal with others it is important that you get this issue of rights sorted out early on.

## The issue of risks and benefits

In keeping a learning journal feelings of discomfort and vulnerability may arise because you are asking yourself questions like, 'why is my clinical practice like this?', 'how did it come to be this way?' and 'how can I improve it?'. A commitment to learn from journal writing is a commitment to a great deal of introspection, honesty with self and a frame of mind that will be able to handle what you come to know in a constructive way. Sharing your journal entries with others may also put at risk such things as your level of self-confidence, call into question aspects of your practice and challenge your much cherished professional values. There are also risks for those who support or facilitate reflection through journal writing like nurse educators, mentors and preceptors. What should or must they do for example if they hear an account of mal-practice or care which the facilitator would consider as unsafe? What happens to notions of trust and confidentiality between people in such circumstances? Who becomes vulnerable, perhaps marginalised or peripheralised? Questions such as 'how far is the account true?', 'how far are we sure of it?' and 'what are the risks associated with not being sure?' need to be asked and responded to (Theobold, 1995).

## The issue of consent

It is important to think through this issue if in your learning journal you are drawing upon the experiences of colleagues as a means to further your own ends. If journal entries are made public and shared for example with peers, issues about who is telling what, to whom and why, need to be sorted out. Additionally the general dialogical environment needs to be supportive of this activity and requires some warmth and collective engagement. In listening to another's account we are given an entrée into someone else's clinical world. In disclosing what is in a learning journal, the 'teller' needs to be sure that they can trust others with what may be a sensitive but certainly a professionally significant issue.

What are some of the 'tensions' that need to be resolved in keeping a learning journal? Earlier we said that a learning journal was comprised of both a content and a process. Now we want to introduce you to the fact that these two elements are held in a 'tensioned' relationship. Some of the most important tensions that need resolving are thus:

### Tension 1: Between writing personal and safe responses

The former is about content. It concerns that which is personally significant to you. The latter combines content with process. It wraps up concerns with what you write about, with the way you write it. Developing your pro-fessionality through journal writing requires the development of an ability to write what you feel needs writing in a fair, accurate and honest manner and often to say things in a critical yet constructive way. Sometimes safe responses are written in a context of fear, dread and blame. Sometimes they are written up so as not to offend if they were to enter the public domain in some way.

### Tension 2: Between nurse-centric and 'significant other' perspectives

This is about using the journal to present your view of things and your ability and preparedness to be open to the views of others. No account is free from bias and an amount of distortion (wilful or unconscious). No account is neutral and impartial. The journal can be used to represent alternative perspectives that allow you to see the same clinical pheno-menon in different ways (Cooper, 1989). It can serve to illuminate the subjective connections of self with significant others (eg. clients, managers, tutors).

### Tension 3: Between privacy and the right to know

This is a complex and very 'contested' issue. We have said

that you have the right to keep the contents of a learning journal private if you so wish. But this raises the moral problem concerning the rights others have to know the content of your journal. Some of these rights are to do with journal writing in a context of professional and organisational accountability. Other rights are more legalistic in kind and relate to the way evidence from a journal might be used in a process of litigation. Then there is the right that some might exercise in terms of 'I have the right to know what it is you are writing about me!'. This is about the right to know and the right to intervene in the light of that information. Rights are problematic because they often contain appeals to different political, professional and moral values (Pring, 1988).

### Tension 4: Between structure and freedom

Sometimes if keeping a learning journal is a pre or post registration course requirement, expectations are raised about how far there is a predetermined structure or format for each entry. Whereas critical incident analysis can be enhanced by certain structured ways of looking and learning from clinical experiences, keeping a learning journal offers health carers the freedom to express themselves in whatever style they choose, unfettered by 'academic' conventions and traditions. In reality a compromise is reached between structuring an entry and the freedom to be creative.

### Tension 5: Between the particular and the general

One journal entry is an account of a particular instance of practice, an encounter, a dialogue, a feeling, an achievement and so on. It is dangerous to read too much into one entry. Journals that contain numerous entries over time provide the potential for generalisation. This might be a generalisation about a personally preferred value position in relation to client care, about a usual way of providing an aspect of care, about a general strategy for managing the busyness of a ward and so on. In this sense 'general' means what you tend to generally do, think and feel. It may or may not be generally true for others. It is important to appreciate the difference between what is generally the case for you and what is not. In reflecting on your journal entries it is also important to try to tease out and establish what is particular and different in certain clinical contexts and what are the more patterned, regular and therefore more general things. If you make these general things known to others, such as peers and work colleagues, you give them the opportunity to generalise from it to their own clinical situation. This is called naturalistic generalisation (Stake, 1995).

### Tension 6: Between dialogue and disillusionment

In some health care contexts extracts from learning journals are shared between peers and with tutors. This is justified on the grounds that learning accrues from the public articulation of the clinical issue and from the dialogue that it generates. The individual has to experience a benefit which might take the form of new perspectives and insights offered by others on 'their issue'. Meaningful dialogues whether in verbal or written form about what has been articulated have to take the individual forward. This sense of moving forward will often be defined in very personal ways. Without this sense, dialogues of this kind can quickly lead to disillusionment and to feelings that the process was a 'waste of time'.

## What are some of the common problems in keeping a learning journal?

Throughout this chapter we have been addressing some of the problems associated with learning journals particularly with their purposes, content and form and the ethical issues that arise from these three things. We want to add four more problems drawn from the work of Paterson (1995) and then leave you, the reader, to weigh up and to counter-balance the pros and cons of learning through journal writing. They are:

1. *The problem of procrastination*: Particularly if it is felt that keeping a learning journal is unworthy of the attention that course work assignments/exams deserve.

2. *The problem of superficial and unreflective entries*: There is no virtue in trying to describe and faithfully regurgitate what has happened to you. The idea is to set out the clinical phenomenon and then to interrogate it through the processes of writing, critical reflection and (in some cases) peer or collegial discussion.

3. *The problem of waning enthusiasm*: To make learning happen it needs to have a chance to take hold and be apprehended. It may help to view the learning journal as a companion, to be committed to make regular entries and re-read them over time.

4. *Unwillingness or inability to reflect*: As we have said earlier, reflection-on-practice is not just a cognitive activity but a moral, affective and ethical art form. You need to read about keeping a learning journal, about reflection being a specialised form of thinking and about learning being a complex activity.

## In what ways can keeping a journal enhance learning?

The learning journal offers a learning experience in several senses. First, there is the opportunity for the health carer to learn more about a substantive aspect of their clinical practice and the organisational culture in which it is embedded. For example, through the journal a nurse might learn more about caring for the elderly, about how to maximise the therapeutic potential of nursing, the rights of the unborn child, effective multidisciplinary team leadership and so on. Secondly, journal writing offers the opportunity to learn about the process of researching clinical practice, what questions to ask, what evidence to gather and what valid claims can be made about improvements in practice. Thirdly, journal writing offers an opportunity to learn about ourselves, about the kind of health care professional we are and wish to be.

For some health care professionals many benefits are claimed from the process of journal writing. In reviewing recent literature the benefits appear to cluster around three domains. Although it is difficult to categorise many of the articles on journal writing the following have something significant to say about the domain with which they have been linked.

(1) *Benefits in the cognitive domain:* about developing specific thinking skills like analysis, evaluation and critical thinking. For example, Hahnemann B (1986) 'Journal Writing: a key to promoting critical thinking in nursing students' and Callister L (1993) 'The Use of Student Journals in Nursing Education: Making Meaning out of Clinical Experience'.

(2) *Benefits in the affective domain*: about feelings, attitudes, emotionality, self concept, confidence and self esteem. For example, Landeen J *et al* (1995) 'Exploring the Lived Experiences of Psychiatric Nursing Students through self-reflective Journals'.

(3) *Benefits in the clinical action/competency domain*: about practical skills, technical competence, strengths and weaknesses. For example, Wallace D (1996) 'Using Reflective Diaries to Assess Students'and Burnard P (1988) 'The Journal as an Assessment and Evaluation Tool in Nurse Education'.

The interesting question that arises from this review is 'why do so few papers refer explicitly to the link between the benefits of journal writing and the **organisational**

**domain**?' One explanation perhaps resides in the commonly held humanistic view that journal writing is essentially a personal activity, for generating self-knowledge that leads to a more enlightened health care professional. This view is associated with professional development residing primarily in the worlds of the technical and the practical. If more was done by nurse educators and others to connect journal writing with critical social theory, the work of Habermas (1971) and emancipatory knowing, then perhaps the role of journal writing that enables health carers to tackle the socio-cultural and politico-economic structures which constrain their lives, could be more widely known and appreciated. Recent research seems to clearly point us in this direction particularly when we read about:

> *'... the often vulnerable and stressed position nurses find themselves in today when trying to meet their professional aspirations within a medically dominated, bureaucratic health-care system.'*
>
> (Graham, 1994: 235)

In our own work, both with nursing students and in particular with those undertaking the ENB 997/998 course, the claims made as a consequence of keeping learning journals are most frequently related to the following:

| Claim 1 | **'It can illuminate my thinking':** | anxieties, prejudices, partial knowledge, mental blocks |
|---|---|---|
| Claim 2 | **'It can show me how open and receptive I am':** | self-disclosure, openness, other points of view |
| Claim 3 | **'I can see how my thinking changes':** | altered appreciations, changing value positions |
| Claim 4 | **'It helps me to appreciate my general attitude to work':** | what I need to work at and improve, my future agenda |

| Claim 5 | 'It helps me get better at what I do': | positive impact on clinical action and the quality of care |
|---|---|---|
| Claim 6 | 'It helps me in my advocacy role': | more able to argue for resources, justify my practice to others, speak on behalf of others |
| Claim 7 | 'It was motivating': | fun to do, compelling once patterns began to emerge, a different thing to do |

# References

Ackoff R (1979) The Future of Operational Research is Past. *Journal of Operational Research Society* **30**: 93–104

Ballantyne R, Packer J (1995) *Making Connections: Using student journals as a Teaching/Learning Aid.* Unpublished paper, School of Professional Studies, Faculty of Education, Queensland University of Technology, Brisbane, Australia.

Berger P, Luckmann T (1976) *The Social Construction of Reality.* Penguin Books, Harmondsworth

Boud D (1996) *Enhancing Learning through Self Assessment.* Kogan Page, London: 14–15

Bowman A (1994) Teaching ethics: telling stories. *Nurse Ed Today* **15** (1): 33–38

Burnard P(1988) The Journal as an Assessment and Evaluation Tool in Nurse Education. *Nurse Ed Today* **8**: 105–107

Burnard P, Chapman C (1993) *Professional and ethical issues in Nursing: The code of professional conduct.* 2nd edition. Scutari, Chichester.

Burnard P, Morrison P (1994) *Nursing Research in Action: Developing Basic Skills.* Macmillan Press, Basingstoke

Callister L (1993) The use of student journals in nursing education: Making meaning out of clinical experience. *J Nurse Ed* **32** (4):185–86

Cooper M (1989) Gilligan's different voice: a perspective for nursing. *J Professional Nurs* **5** (1):10–16

Department of Health (1989a) *Education and Training; working paper ten.* HMSO, London

Department of Health (1989b) *Working for Patients.* HMSO, London

Department of Health (1993) *A Vision for the Future.* NHS Management Executive

English National Board (1991) *Framework for Continuing Professional Education for Nursing, Midwifery and Health Visiting: Guide to Implementation.* ENB, London

English National Board (1994) *Creating Lifelong Learners: Partnerships for Care.* ENB, London

Ghaye T *et al*(1996a) *Theory-Practice Relationships: Reconstructing Practice.* Pentaxion Ltd, Newcastle upon Tyne

Ghaye T *et al*(1996b) *Professional Values: Being a Professional.* Pentaxion Ltd, Newcastle upon Tyne

Graham I (1994) How do registered nurses think and experience nursing: A phenomenological investigation. *J Clinical Nurs* **3**: 235–242

Guba E, Lincoln Y (1989) *Fourth Generation Evaluation.* Sage Publications, London.

Habermas J (1971) *Knowledge and Human Interests.* Beacon, Boston.

Hahnemann B (1986) Journal writing: A key to promoting critical thinking in nursing students. *J Nurs Ed* **25**: 213–15

Holly ML (1987) *Keeping a personal-professional journal.* Deakin University Press, Victoria

Holly ML (1989) *Writing to Grow: Keeping a Personal-Professional Journal.* Heinemann, Portsmouth, NH

Landeen J *et al* (1995) Exploring the lived experiences of psychiatric nursing students through self-reflective journals. *J Adv Nurs* **21**: 878–885

McNiff J (1990) Writing and the creation of educational knowledge. In: Lomax P (Ed) *Managing Staff Development in Schools.* Multi-Lingual Matters, Clevedon: 56

Paterson B (1995) Developing and maintaining reflection in

clinical journals. *Nurse Ed Today* **15**: 211–220

Pring R (1988) Confidentiality and the right to know. In: Murphy R, Torrance H (Eds) (1988) *Evaluating Education: Issues and Methods*. Paul Chapman, London

Stake R (1995) *The Art of Case Study Research*. Sage Publications, London

Theobold M (1995) *The Nature of Nursing Knowledge*. Keynote speech at the Conference on Reflective Practice: The Impact on Patient Care, Commonwealth Institute, London

Thomas D (1992) *Putting Nature to the Rack: Narrative Studies as Research*. Paper presented at the Teacher's Stories of Life and Work Conference, Chester, UK

Wallace D (1996) Using Reflective Diaries to assess students. *Nurs Standard*, **10** (36): 44–47

# 4

# Examples of journal writing

In chapter 3 we raised the question, 'what do I put into a learning journal?' In this chapter we have included some examples of the different ways health care professionals have made their journal entries. Above all other things each entry must be:

- Concerned with something professionally significant

- Written or entered in your journal in such a way that it makes sense to you.

There is no real virtue in trying to follow some notions of 'academic convention' each time you use your journal. You must create the kind of 'text' that we described earlier. This is a 'text' that you can learn from. There are no 'writing rules'. You should let go of any notions that you have of trying to 'get it right first time'. The personal relevance and meaningfulness of your journal entries are important qualities. So in keeping a journal you should not get bogged down with issues of 'better' or 'worse', about writing better, tighter, more economically, having more control of words because this begs the tricky question, 'what constitutes better?' More important is trying to create entries which allow you to search for new angles on professional concerns, biases, fragmented and woolley thinking, new juxtapositions and important associations that perhaps had remained unknown to you and been uncelebrated. It is also important to avoid the 'paralysis by analysis syndrome'. Be patient and realistic with what you want to get out of your journal writing. It is unrealistic to think that new, wonderful clinical insights will emerge, as if by magic, from one or two short entries!

In making a journal entry, what you focus upon and how you record it are two things that need to be thought through. For example, in making a conscious decision to focus upon those aspects of your work that are professionally significant, you may focus upon one thing such as your 'decision making', or your 'inter-personal skills' or your ability to 'develop shared beliefs and understandings' within a team. Alternatively you may feel that you want to focus upon lots of different things that are professionally significant. Both approaches are legitimate. Both have two things in common. First you need to create a number of 'texts'. That is to say you need to make multiple entries, over time. This relates to the issue of giving yourself a chance to let the 'problematics' of your clinical practice come to the surface. Secondly the texts you create need to be interrogated at a later date. It is through this process of interrogation that learning from reflection-on-practice can begin to take a hold. In keeping a learning journal there must be a commitment on your part to return to the 'texts' that you have created and to learn from them. Learning arises from the re-exploration of past experiences. You may get caught up in the swirl of so many things that you might give your attention to. A more unified, consistent and holistic understanding of practice can be a struggle but it should be your goal.

In this chapter we identify six examples of 'types of journal entry'. Each type represents a different way of re-presenting what the health carer wanted to record in their journal. Sometimes a series of entries in your journal might be in the same form. But there is no reason why you should not change the form of your entry in the same way that you might change the focus of it. One entry might also embrace more than one form. The 'types of journal entry' that are most often used we have labelled thus:

- Faithful regurgitation type
- Off-load type
- Extend and revise type
- Concept mapping type
- Knotty and messy type
- Living contradiction type.

What follows are some examples of each type. In publishing these we have had to be mindful of the issues of consent and confidentiality. We have sampled from a range of types of entry. We have also had permission to edit each one so that their main characteristic comes through clearly. However, there is a natural blurring of the edges between types.

## Example 1: The faithful regurgitation type

The emphasis in entries of this kind is upon 'what I've done'. They tend to be mainly descriptive and can be written up in a vivid manner. There is a reflective component and sometimes an evaluative dimension. There is often an initial anxiety in relation to 'will this entry tell me anything later'. There can also be problems with selection, detail and length of the entry. Sometimes the entry takes on the air of a pseudo and mini-essay. Sometimes such entries contain references to the professional and/or medical literature. The example is from an experienced paediatric nurse who is keeping a journal as part of an award-bearing continuing professional development course. She has just spent the day in seminar work discussing HIV infection and AIDS in children.

'Well we started the day on time...thank goodness because if we had started late again all the seminars would have got behind. Trudy and Julie gave the first presentation...they were really good, dynamic, confident...all the kinds of thing that I hoped mine would be. It's better I think if you do it together....but I drew the short straw so had to do it on my own. Trudy and Julie spoke a lot about the American research. I couldn't believe that 1,500–2,000 HIV-infected infants can be expected to be born each year in the States! They finished well in talking about issues of vulnerability and dependency because of the nature of the disease and its social context.

I was quite pleased with my presentation. I kept to time...45 minutes is not enough though. I got through the things I wanted to say. I even used the overhead and got the acetates the right way around for a change! I made my three main points about children being infected with HIV through three main routes: (a) receipt of infected blood, (b) sexual or drug use behaviours or, (c) vertical transmission from an infected mother. It seemed to go alright. There weren't many questions at the end...but they did seem interested. I was quite nervous....and maybe I might have slowed down what I said. I think they got a bit over-loaded...they were interested though...I think.'

## Example 2: The off-load type

Entries of this kind tend to be high on emotionality with the nurse often claiming that the entry is 'personal and pertinent'. They often focus upon an encounter with significant others, often colleagues and can contain disagreements over practice and/or policy. The entry is 'significant' in that it makes us cross, it will not go away, has not resolved itself or has questioned our professionality. Some entries of this type can be quite judgemental. The writing process can be cathartic. Through it we can purge ourselves of pent up emotions (Holly, 1989). The example is from the journal of a nurse who is working with a psychiatric patient.

'Oh my goodness what a day...I sometimes wonder why I do this work. It's hard enough without all this. Why is it that he (the doctor) always treats me like an idiot. He knows best.. he just doesn't seem to listen. It's not that I am questioning his ability or even his judgement....but I do know Jim (the patient)...I know him bloody well. Jim has been telling me that he feels that the drugs are making him feel unwell...he has said this for some time. I try to tell the doctor this but he thinks that Jim's condition will get worse if the drugs are discontinued. All I want is to be taken seriously.....I don't feel that I am being listened to. I can't seem to speak to the doctor in the right way. I can't find the right reply to what that person says! Jim can't argue for himself so I've got to do it for him. Jim has rights...I have rights...why won't he seem to listen?'

## Example 3: The extend and revise type

This type can only be found in journals where the nurse has made a number of entries and it comes into being through revisiting, reviewing and re-appreciating earlier entries. It is evidence of a systematic and committed approach to reflect-on-practice. With entries of this kind there is an opportunity to do a number of things such as:

(a)   Celebrate the good and rewarding aspects of practice

(b)   Continue to moan about the bad bits of your work

(c)   Re-relieve yourself of any feelings of frustration

(d)   Remind yourself of the things that you had forgotten

(e)   Re-examine earlier responses to significant incidents

(f)   Look again for beliefs, prejudices and those things that get in the way of moving your practice forward

(g) Separate out in your head those things that you have some control over and can influence from those that you presently cannot

(h) Take stock of 'where you are at'.

In adopting this style it is important to date each entry. In this way you will be able to place altered or confirmed thoughts, feelings and actions on a time line. This temporal dimension to your journal entries might give you a way in to understanding more richly notions of professional 'development'. The example is drawn from the journal of a nurse who is working with children with profound and multiple learning difficulties. Early in her journal she develops some 'brief sketches' of the children with whom she works most closely.

### Date: September

*'John*

Aged 9. John sits quietly and passively in his wheelchair. He 'comes alive' when placed on the floor, moving about by lively actions which are neither rolling nor crawling. John is unable to travel in any particular direction and has no sense of danger and therefore wears a safety helmet. He cannot walk. John does not appear to use gesture of any sort to indicate his understanding or needs and cannot speak. He often appears impervious to stimulation but occasionally shows real pleasure by looking intently at some wind-chimes or some disco-type lighting. John is unable to feed himself and is doubly incontinent and severely epileptic.

*James*

James is 9 and cortically blind but walks with help and splashes around the swimming pool with armbands. James can communicate and although his speech is limited and repetitive he makes relationships with his carers. James needs...and demands...a great deal of attention. He explores the environment with his hands but is unaware of his own strength, cheerfully destroying playthings. James needs help to feed himself with a spoon. He is doubly incontinent and epileptic.

*Jayne*

7 years old and unable to speak, Jayne often looks around at everything and everyone with interest. She has a beautiful smile and is able to communicate to a very limited degree by facial expressions and sounds. Jayne is unable to walk. She has difficulty in using her hands but enjoys being helped to play with toys. Jayne is at the early stages of learning to feed herself. She is incontinent.

## Date: May the next year

These sketches of the children were among the first entries in my journal...the first pieces of reflective writing. I have often read them over but always uncritically. But now I am returning to them with some distress. I feel the descriptions are negative and mechanistic...The terms used reflect my deep steeping in medical models of care and negative attitudes towards children with PMLD. On reflection, the sketches are an unfortunate entrée to my journal. The following is a second attempt at James' sketch:

James is a handsome boy from a very warm and loving family. Despite blindness and disabilities due to an early childhood illness he has learned to speak. He frequently delights us with things that he says (often single words) which show that he has understood the situation. He has a wicked sense of fun and a 'party spirit'. When working with James you have to be careful not to let him know you would like him to do X. It is better to approach things in a 'sidelong' manner or he will insist on doing Y instead, usually grinning as he does so! James has an attractive personality which people 'take to' and therefore he generally gets plenty of attention...which he thrives on. James enjoys himself a lot and gives pleasure to many people.

This sketch offers, I think, a more rounded 'human' picture. It provides a vivid contrast to my earlier writing particularly as I've decided to write on the opposite page. Again, however, the picture is limited and distorted compared with the full complexity of this child. It also seems fairly patronising and does not attempt a look at James' views on the world. This in turn may say quite a lot about my world view! These are issues I will need to explore later in my journal.'

## Example 4: The concept mapping type

Entries of this type are increasing in their popularity. They are more pictorial or 'graphical' than literary. A concept map contains health care knowledge which is represented in the form of a labelled-line graph structure in which the three fundamental elements are:

- *Nodes*: these are key ideas or concepts
- *Links*: these are lines drawn between the nodes
- *Relations*: this is the meaning given to the nodes by the nature of the links. between them. In essence concept maps, as journal entries, are personal reality maps, constructed by you, to express the sense or meaning you currently have of a particular facet of your health care work. They are your subjective construction of an aspect of your world. If your journal contains a number of maps which focus on the same area or issue, then learning can arise because their analysis can reveal how:

  * you might fine tune 'know that', 'know how' and your 'know why' knowledge

  * far ideas remain isolated or more integrated and structured in your mind

  * you may have changed your perception of aspects of your practice over time.

Figure 10 shows an example of a concept map where a nurse is reflecting upon some of the 'building blocks' for professional development. Notice how she has placed 'reflection' in the centre of her map and the questioning tone that the map conveys.

## Example 5: The knotty and messy type

'Knots' have been described by Wagner (1987) as the inter-relationship between cognitive and affective processes which lead to conflict and professional dilemmas. Drawing upon theories in cognitive psychology, clinical psychology and psychotherapy she identifies six types of conflicts or 'knots', some of which might be short lived, others lasting for years. What each type of 'knot' has in common is that they arise due to a discrepancy or dilemma between 'what is' and 'what must or should be'. Ackoff (1979) uses the notion of 'messes' to express a similar kind of thing. In our everyday clinical practice our thinking often gets snarled up in a 'knot'. Knots can effect our clinical action. Sometimes we react to knots by complaining. Knots need tackling. The example is drawn from the journal of an experienced neonatal nurse who has been given the role of establishing a 'nursing development unit' (NDU). The 'knot' is centrally about re-defining and clarifying roles.

> 'I really feel under some pressure. I'm still not sure of my role... its blurring a lot with that of ward sister. I'm not sure how far I should keep some clinical involvement, retreat from ward activity... just get on with the strategic and business bit. I feel pretty screwed up right now because I haven't resolved how I should... or must... try to balance clinical care with my managerial responsibilities. I want to avoid being too "distant" though.... I guess I've got to sort out some kind of balance between my clinical and developmental commitments. I can speak the language of clinical practice but can I speak the language of management sufficiently well?... Its something I've got to

unravel and sort out.'

**Figure 10.**

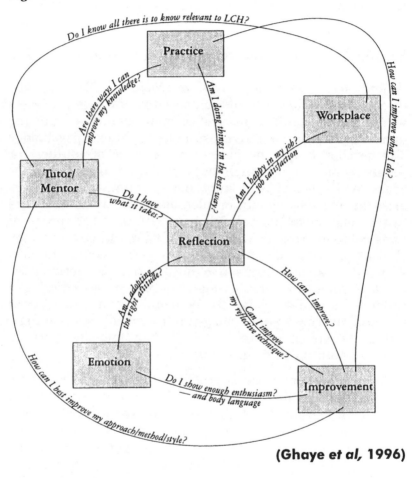

(Ghaye *et al,* 1996)

## Example 6: The living contradiction type

Journal entries of this type acknowledge that clinical practice is a value-laden activity. The entries focus upon the nature of the professional values that give clinical practice its shape, form and purpose. A prerequisite for being able to write entries of this kind is knowing your professional values. The entry then focuses upon how far you are able to live out your values in your practice. The extent to which you are able to do this and support such a claim are important entries to make. It is also important to record those things which enable and facilitate this process and also the impediments. Additionally there is an opportunity for you to focus your attention on the 'contradictions' (Whitehead, 1994) in your clinical work. A contradiction can be those occasions when we say one thing and yet act in a manner which is inconsistent and which contradicts that espoused value position. If we take Whitehead's suggestion to consider ourselves as 'living contradictions' we can write about these, over time, and regard them as professional growth points. It is not a question of trying to eradicate all contradictions from our practice, our professional lives are not as straightforward as this. With some contradictions we may have to say to ourselves, 'well I've been exploring this through my journal writing for some time now and I've come to the conclusion that that's how it is and there isn't a great deal I can do about things for the time being'. The examples are drawn from a number of individual journals from nurses and midwives. They all reflect contradictions between what people say and do.

> 'I believe that a patient's quality of life is the most important consideration, and yet I use sophisticated technology which prolongs a life which has no future, purpose and happiness, and more suffering is caused by a continuance.

> I believe that I should always take the time and care to answer a patient's questions fully and unhurriedly and yet due to the pressure of being a ward co-ordinator, I am not always able to do this.

> I believe that each patient that I am responsible for is worthy of my constant care and attention because each one has mental health problems unique to them and

needs "professional" attention... and yet... time and re-sources prevent this, resulting in nurses being involved in intensive care or crisis management with people with less "risky/acute" problems taking a back seat.

I believe parents should be allowed to stay with their children in our department at all times, but because some consultants do not allow this, I am always asking parents to go, so I am always in conflict. Parents have rights.'

These examples of journal writing reflect the different ways health care professionals have tried to sharpen their perceptions of the everyday realities of their clinical work. Journal writing can help us to extend our understandings, insights and command of the clinical situations in which we work. These examples have shown that keeping a journal can help us to recognise contradictions of purpose and value. The examples represent authentic portrayals of clinical experience. They are 'realities' which need to be constructed, deconstructed, interrogated, critiqued and transformed over time. One nurse wrote about this process in a most vivid manner.

'...all the turning back and turning over, and again. I felt I was pushing myself into corners and forcing myself to stay there until I'd worked out a valid response or answer to things. And then it got worse as I took it more seriously. Back in the corners again and this time instead of crawling around muttering, I felt I had to stand up and confront the corners. I did feel like bumping around in the dark. Then it began to dawn on me. I was refusing to see that it was me who had to switch on the lights. And the switches... Generally... were just above my head. In the end I found some interesting pictures in the corners and it made a real change from circling around in the middle of the room.'

These examples emphasise the importance of concentrating on particularity and our everyday clinical experiences in our search for new knowledge, understandings and sensitivities.

In turning to the new science of chaos we find ample support for this belief.

*'The modern study of chaos began with the creeping realisation in the 1960s that quite simple mathematical equations could model systems every bit as violent as a waterfall. Tiny differences in input could quickly become overwhelming differences in output... In weather, for example, this translates into what is only half-jokingly known as the butterfly effect — the notion that a butterfly stirring the air today in Peking can transform storm systems next month in New York.'*

(Gleick, 1988: 8)

The entries we place in our learning journals is knowledge encapsulated in particularity. In the stirrings of these butterfly wings we have the starting point for transforming our understanding about the nature of our professionalism and for improving the quality of client care.

# References

Ackoff R (1979) The Future of Operational Research is Past. *J Operational Research Society* **30** (2): 93–104

Ghaye T (1996) *Professional Values: being a professional.* Pentaxion Press, Newcastle upon Tyne

Gleick J (1988) *Making a New Science.* Heinemann, New York

Holly ML (1989) *Writing to Grow: Keeping a Personal-Professional Journal.* Heinemann, Portsmouth, NH

Wagner A (1987) 'Knots' in Teacher's Thinking. In: Calderhead J (Ed) (1987) *Exploring Teacher's Thinking.* Cassell Education, London

Whitehead J (1994) *Creating Living Educational Theory.* Hyde Publications, Bournemouth, UK

# 5

# Critical incident analysis

Minghella and Benson (1995) identify that critical incident analysis has been espoused as a valuable method of promoting reflective practice in nursing and it can be used as a tool in developing curriculum content. Benner (1984) also notes the use of critical incident analysis and its assistance in attaining competence in nursing skills and the development of the 'expert practitioner'. Powell (1989) noted that experienced practice is not wholly dependent upon the time spent in the job, therefore the experience has to be gained through some other process. Critical incident analysis can be used as one of those processes that assist the individual in becoming an experienced practitioner.

In this chapter we will attempt to explore the use and value of using critical incident analysis and its identification of learning through experience, thereby moving forward the professional boundaries and promoting 'good' practice.

Critical incident analysis may also be used as a tool to develop and identify reflective practice for individual practitioners, providing them with a means of keeping records of evidence for their personal professional profile and so fulfiling part of the PREP requirements.

It is advocated by Parker *et al* (1995) that through using critical incidents, the development of knowledge, skills and attitudes are grounded in practice by means of reflection on action. This chapter will also attempt to guide the individual practitioner in the identification and recording of critical incidents, discussing the value of experiential learning and gaining new knowledge through their practice. The recording of these incidents may also act as a measure of the individual's practice fulfilling both the professional and governmental requirements of clinical practice discussed in chapters 1 and 7.

## Where do critical incidents come from?

John Flannagan (1954), an aviation psychologist with the United States Air Force, developed the procedure for gathering information concerning effective and ineffective behaviour in certain situations. The combat veterans whom he was studying reported incidents which they considered either helpful or inadequate in accomplishing a designated mission. Flannagan produced a focused description that provided a systematic, open ended procedure for obtaining data in both a verbal or written format. He then analysed these incidents and produced a list of critical behaviours for the performance of tasks. It was Benner (1984) who primarily introduced them into nursing and suggested that they would assist in the development of expertise in nursing.

Using critical incidents Benner suggests that over a period of time, following exposure to theory, and reflection on its application to clinical practice, they will assist the individual practitioner to develop what she refers to as an 'expert practitioner'. Benner notes that the theory taught in the basic training of nurses offers knowledge that can be made explicate and formalised, this is the 'scientific knowledge' described by Carper (1978). Benner refers to it as concrete theory or the science of nursing. Clinical practice, however, she notes is more complex and presents many more realities for the individual practitioner than can be captured by scientific knowledge alone. Benner notes that what she refers to as the 'expert practitioner' can be influenced through this process providing positive outcomes for the practitioner's clients. Clinical knowledge, argues Schon (1987) develops as practical experience which is combined with the application of theoretical knowledge and is further redefined and extended with practice. Schon (1983) recommended reflection on critical incidents as a valuable learning tool. Flannagan's critical incident technique has also been used in nursing to elicit indicators of high and low quality of nursing care (Norman *et al*, 1992).

Critical incidents may then assist the individual practitioner in drawing on their experience, helping them to make sense of those experiences, facilitating learning through them and allowing them to utilise their scientific knowledge applying it to clinical practice. Chesney (1996) argues that reflecting on past experiences and making sense of them assists in the application of theory to practice; this being the scientific knowledge applied into clinical practice.

## What are critical incidents?

Critical incidents are defined as:

> *'incidents happen, but critical incidents are produced by the way we look at a situation, it is an interpretation of the significance of the event.'*
>
> (Tripp. 1993: 8)

or described as:

> *'Snapshot views of daily work of the nurse and by examining them the effects of care on patients can be seen, and interactions between colleagues can be highlighted.'*
>
> (Clamp, 1980: 1756)

Critical incidents are not therefore just the experiences we all live through, but experiences we analyse and use to identify aesthetic knowledge and the experiential learning acquired. It is the analysis and evaluation of the experience that can then be used to improve clinical practice, apply scientific knowledge and ultimately develop and provide evidence of an 'expert practitioner'.

In the health care arena the word 'critical' often conjures up an experience that has had some major implications on our practice or an incident of an emergency nature, ie. cardiac arrest or drug error. Although these situations can be used as critical incidents and learning experiences they are not the only experiences that can be used. Any experience that the individual encounters is potentially a critical incident and therefore a situation the individual can reflect upon.

The actual incident can then be:

- An incident that is an ordinary experience
- An incident where the experience did not go to plan (these may be positive as well as negative experiences)
- An incident that went well
- An incident that reflects the values and beliefs held by the individual
- An incident that identifies the contribution of qualified practitioners
- An incident that allows the identification of learning.

Minghella and Benson (1995) note in their study that most incidents appear to represent interpersonal or interactional situations rather than clinical procedural problems: the latter is also a valuable tool to identify our practice.

It is the reflection on these incidents and the analysis of these that assist the practitioner in moving their practice forward and obtaining the expert nurse status.

# How to find an incident

We experience new and repeated incidents every day of our lives; the practice we now perform has often been learnt from previous experiences. The problem with this experiential learning so far is that it has not been at a conscious level or recorded in any form as required by PREP (UKCC, 1990). So how do we identify an incident for ourselves that will demonstrate our professional knowledge and competence and assist in providing a good quality of care to our clients?

Some of these incidents can be drawn from past experiences where the experience made an impact on our practice.

'As a student I remember my first death. This was a critical incident that some 18 years later I can remember vividly. The situation was on a care of the elderly ward and I was to assist the qualified nurse in the laying out procedure. The nurse explained what we were to do and allowed me to talk through the procedure before going into the patient. The two of us then proceeded to lay the patient out maintaining dignity and respect for the deceased. Following the procedure the nurse again talked through what we had done and my feelings related to the task. This incident is still recalled as I review my own approach to the laying out of clients, the way I was treated had influenced how I wanted to assist individuals in their first encounters with the dead patient. It was a positive incident that I could reflect upon and so inform my practice, through the experience learning together with the scientific knowledge taught in the classroom, this provided me with an example of good nursing practice.'

Equally these experiences happen to us in our current practice and can have as just much effect on the way we deliver our care. Alternatively, on the way home from work we often think back on the day's activities, the situations that have arisen and how we dealt with them. These can be as important to our practice as the major events and, if recorded, will provide a rich source of reflection that can then be consciously analysed.

Recording these incidents is important. The longer they are left the less easy it is to record the detail necessary to conduct a proper evaluation of them. They may initially be recorded in the learning journal as discussed in chapters 3 and 4.

## How to analyse the incident

These incidents can be used to offer a starting point for self examination of our values, beliefs and self understanding, as well as written evidence for the professional requirements. Tripp (1993) suggests that in analysing these events we may be able to verify something we suspected or reveal something entirely new.

Tripp identifies five methods of analysing the incidents. These are:

- Thinking strategies

- The Why? challenge

- The dilemma identification

- Personal theory analysis

- Ideology critique.

### Thinking strategies

Tripp (1993) uses certain thinking strategies to assist in the analysis of the identified incident. He suggests that framing questions about the incidents can lead us to a deeper reading or seeking of scientific knowledge on the subject encountered. The care of the patient with a new condition or the administration of a new drug could be overlooked by practitioners if they were merely to look after the patient;the thinking strategy analysing their practice will provide the individuals with the ability to seek further scientific and other types of knowledge that may then have an effect on the care that they administer.

Tripp (1993) also suggests that this thinking strategy should take the form of reviewing the non event, in other words what did not happen. If a situation went well it is not in our nature to question or to think about it again. In this analysis Tripp suggests that we review what may have happened rather than continuing our practice blindly. What if it had happened in a different way? It may have been better. Or, if something had not happened, how can we be assured this was not just by chance? To continue good practice we also need to reflect on the positive incidents and the things to celebrate in our practice. These are just as 'critical' and need to be nourished. The value of looking at practice and the same situation from other points of view, utilising the knowledge that we have gained over time, can sometimes illuminate different perspectives on the same aspect of care. These new ways of seeing may provide useful ways to take our practice forward.

## The Why? challenge

Tripp suggests that if we continue to ask why-type questions of our practice, we will often end up with one of two answers. The first is, *'because that is how it ought to be'*. This assists in recognising that we are operating from deeply held beliefs. For example, what if we ask, 'Why do you wash patients rather than letting them do it for themselves?' Through an analysis of this it may be possible to identify the individual's belief in nursing that they are there to do this for the patients. The second answer is often, *'because that is how it is'*. Tripp argues that this denotes something we take for granted and therefore feel we cannot change.

'I remember when on the wards the patients temperatures were taken every four hours even as they left to go home, if I had been asked why at the time, I probably would have replied in the above manner after justifying the importance of temperature taking and all the arguments that I could have thought of.'

This approach of the why challenge may lead us into exploring new alternatives or identifying areas for future practitioner research.

## Dilemma identification

This is another useful way to make sense of practice. Our clinical work is full of dilemmas. They often present themselves as mis-matches between what we say and do, think and feel, between our values-in-practice and those of others. As one professional holds differing beliefs from another we can be faced with some dilemma in judgement or decision-making, for instance, the doctor who does not want the patient to know their diagnosis as against the patient who trusts in you and asks what is wrong with them. Where do we go for help? Who are we accountable to? What about the nurse's professional judgement? How do these incidents provide a means of learning from and the promotion of 'good practice'? The first step is to recognise and appreciate that there is a dilemma present in our practice. Once this has been identified the process of critical reflection and meaning-making can begin.

## Personal theory analysis

Here Tripp argues that we need to articulate our set of beliefs that are informing our professional judgement and thereby our action in the material world, for example do we believe 'nursing' is doing for the patient or assisting the patient? Both beliefs will result in slightly different care being given to the clients. Choosing one solution over the other enables us to identify the values that we hold inherent in our professional judgement. Analysis may identify for us where our personal theory is grounded and therefore why we practice in the manner demonstrated.

## Ideology critique

Tripp argues that this process has to do with the way in which certain ideas represent the world to us. This makes us behave and think in certain ways to legitimise what we do or have done to us by others, so providing a rationale for our behaviour. Ideologies are big, organising frameworks that have political, professional and personal aspects to them and thus are harder to analyse than the more specific and practice-based examples already given.

# Recording critical incidents

There are several formats that can be used to record the process of critical incident analysis (Benner, 1984; Minghella and Benson, 1995; Lillyman and Evans, 1996). The idea of recording and analysing these incidents can, for example, be used as evidence for the PREP requirements, for use at job interviews and to demonstrate learning through practice.

It is suggested for the purpose of the profile that the incident and analysis is limited to one side of A4 (see Figure 11) and that the description preserves the anonymity of those involved and the clinical context. The analysis should always stipulate the learning that has accrued and its application and relevance for practice. Chapter 6 provides a number of incidents that can be analysed in a variety of ways.

**Figure 11: Lillyman and Evans (1996)**

| Critical incident analysis |
|---|
| Description of the incident? |
| By whom was it handled? |
| What learning occurred? |
| What were the outcomes of this incident? |
| How has this incident affected your practice? |

To recap, there are several reasons why critical incident analysis is useful to the practitioner:

1.    As mentioned it provides for the practitioner the evidence required to enter into their professional profile for the PREP requirements and provides evidence of professional development.

2.    It can provide the individual with incidents of good practice that can be used at an interview situation to identify the interaction of theory with practice and/or how practice has been adapted, enriched and improved through reflection.

3.    It provides the individual with written evidence and records of their professional development as they move through their career and gain more experiential knowledge through their practice.

4.    It provides evidence of an ability to 'theorise' about practice which is a quality needed for enrolment on award-bearing courses or to gain some accreditation of prior experiential learning.

5.    It provides evidence which may help us to identify the reflective practitioner in the clinical environment.

6.    It provides evidence of the unique contribution that health care professionals can make in the clinical situation.

7.    The analysis of critical incidents can also be viewed as rich, contextual research data to add fuel to the argument that health care should be and is evidence-based.

Critical incident analysis is then primarily for the individual practitioner to facilitate their professional development and identify and justify changes in their practice.

# References

Benner P (1984) *From Novice to Expert*. Addison Wesley, California

Carper B (1978) Fundamental Patterns of Knowing. *Adv Nurs Sci* **1**: 13–23

Chesney M (1996) Sharing Reflections on Critical Incidents in Midwifery Practice. *Brit J Midwifery* **4** (1): 8–10

Clamp C (1980) Learning through Incidents. *Nurs Times* Oct 2: 1755–1758

Dewey J (1933) *How We Think*. Henrey Regney, Chicago

Flannagan J (1954) The Critical Incident Technique. *Psychol Bull* **51**: 327–358

Lillyman S, Evans B (1996) *Designing a Personal Portfolio/Profile: A workbook for healthcare professionals*. Quay Books, Mark Allen Publishing Group, Dinton, Salisbury, Wiltshire

Minghella E, Benson A (1995) Developing Reflective Practice in Mental Health Nursing Through Critical Incident Analysis. *J Adv Nurs* **21**: 205–213

Norman I, Redfern S, Tomlin D, Oliver S (1992) Developing Flannagan's Critical Incident Technique to Elicit Indicators of High and Low Quality Nursing Care. *J Adv Nurs* **17**: 590–600

Parker D, D'Souza B, Webb J (1995) The value of critical Incident Analysis as an Educational Tool and its Relationship to Experiential Learning. *Nurse Ed Today* **15**: 111–116

Powell J (1989) The Reflective Practitioner in Nursing. *J Adv Nurs* **14**: 824–832

Schon D (1983) *The Reflective Practitoner: How Practitioners Think in Action*. Harper Collins, San Francisco

Schon D (1987) *Educating the Reflective Practitioner*. Jossey Bass, San Francisco

Tripp D (1993) *Critical Incidents in Teaching*. Routledge, London: 8

UKCC (1990) The Report of Post Registration Education and Practice Project. UKCC, London

UKCC (1992) Professional Code of Conduct. UKCC, London

# 6

# Examples of critical incident analysis

The following chapter will provide several examples of critical incident analysis identifying how and where these can be applied to clinical practice. The examples are provided as guidelines to help to identify learning and do not necessarily identify an expert practitioner. The incidents analysed in this chapter may be used in personal professional profiles as evidence of the development of expertise in clinical practice. They can identify where the aesthetic knowledge has been acquired through an individual's clinical practice and experience. Critical incident analysis recognises that learning occurs outside the formal boundaries of academic study and therefore promotes the idea of the health care professional as a life long learner.

## Uses of critical incident analysis in personal profiles

Critical incident analysis can be used in various personal profiles that individual practitioners will produce in their careers, these include the profile for:

- Job interviews
- Accreditation of prior experiential learning

- Post Registration Education and Practice Requirements (PREP).

## Job interviews

Critical incident analysis can be used in the preparation for a job interview. When putting a profile together it is suggested that the profile reflects the job description/person specification for the job. The individual may then draw on their experiences in practice to analyse how they dealt with a given situation (see example 1), identifying how theory and practice interrelate.

## Post Registration Education and Practice Project (PREP)

The PREP requirements (UKCC,1990) provide an ideal opportunity to utilise critical incident analysis. They may be used in the personal professional profile to identify how the individual has maintained and developed in their clinical competence. The analysis of the incident provides a written format stating how personal and practice knowledge interact with the clinical context. Critical incident analysis can also be used as a developmental measurement tool. Here the individual practitioner can, over time, measure their personal and professional development in their clinical practice and identify where and how it has changed, for instance the analysis may identify how the individual deals with an issue today compared to a similar experience earlier in their career. The analysis may then explain why their practice has changed in relation to acquiring new scientific and experiential knowledge, gaining expertise in their field of practice and/or due to the introduction of new policies and procedures (see example 2).

## Accreditation of prior experiential learning (APEL)

On entering courses or gaining accreditation for prior

learning the profile plays a valid part in the analysis and assessment of practice. Critical incident analysis can be used here to reflect on the learning that has occurred in clinical practice and how the individual has utilised theory in their area of practice, identifying areas of specialist and advanced practice (see example 3).

## Recording critical incidents

It is suggested when using critical incidents in profiles for job interviews and PREP requirements that the incident analysis be limited to one side of A4. This will assist those reading it to gain an overview of the learning that has occurred. For *APEL* the word limit is usually set by the institution you are seeking accreditation with and guidelines must be gained from that institution prior to completing the profile.

## Critical incident analysis used for job interviews

Example 1 identifies an incident analysed in a way so that it could be incorporated into a profile for a job interview. The incident discussed in this example was used for a job interview where the nurse was seeking to move from an adult to a paediatric oncology ward. On reviewing the job description the post would expect the individual to have some knowledge and experience in caring for a dying child and the support required for the whole family. This nurse, when applying for this post, did not have any first hand experience specifically with the dying child as all her experience to date was with the dying adult. Although some skills she noted were transferable from the care of the adult patient, the situation was somewhat different in its contextual and emotional issues. As the nurse had no first hand experience she reflected on her training where she had worked on the paediatric wards, observing qualified practitioners who dealt with the dying child. The nurse described a situation that she had observed as a student. The incident was then analysed with the specific job description in mind for a specific interview.

When attending the interview the nurse was then able to discuss the incident and learning that occured as she was questioned about her ability and skills in dealing with the dying child. She was not able in this situation to use her own practice, but identified an area of what she perceived as good practice from the observation of the qualified nurse dealing with the situation. She then analysed the experience and noted why she perceived it as 'good' practice informing the panel at the interview of what she had learnt from her observations and how she would utilise the knowledge gained from her observations when facing the situation for herself.

## Example 1: Critical Incident Analysis

### Description of incident:

'While working on a paediatric medical ward there were several occasions where I was able to observe a staff nurse and her approach to the dying child and relatives. Relationships with the patients and their family played an important part of the process. On the day the child died the staff nurse on duty allocated her time to the child making sure that she was responsible for talking with the relatives, allowing them space and time to grieve, offering support without being over bearing.'

### By whom was it handled?

'This incident was handled by the staff nurse who had built up a relationship with the family and the patient. Each death where possible in this clinical area was handled in the same manner.'

### What learning occurred?

'For me it was the building up of the relationship and the

preparation for the expected death that played a major role in dealing with the situation. Supporting all involved throughout the illness and then follow up. The grieving process could be identified in this situation from the time of diagnosis and observing the staff nurse as she recognised and supported the relatives through the various stages even when stages of grief were repeated as the time went on.'

## What were the outcomes of the incident?

'It was observing an holistic approach for the patient and their family, the importance of clear communication between all the multidisciplinary team as they came into contact with the people involved. Working within a team and recognising and reacting appropriately to the grieving process.'

## How has this incident affected your practice?

'The incident has demonstrated to me the difference in dealing with the dying child and the adult and highlighted the areas where skills are transferable in each situation.'

## Analysing example 1

For this critical incident a thinking strategy was applied in the analysis of the experience. The analysis was on the observation of another professional's practice. The nurse was able to draw on learning from the situation and then analyse the practice to identify how she would deal with a similar situation in her own practice. The incident allowed the nurse to reflect on the scientific knowledge that she had been taught in the classroom, ie. theory relating to care of the dying patient and the importance of good communication skills, caring in an holistic way and support for the relatives as they go through the grieving process before and following the death of the child. The incident included other issues that were relevant to this situation, for example the importance of team work within the clinical environment and the role of the multidisciplinary team in the care of the dying child. Using Tripps' (1993) analysis of critical incidents certain thinking strategies had been used in this situation as the incident allowed the observer to reflect on the incident and apply scientific knowledge to practice, identifying gaps in that knowledge that may require further study or research. In this case gaps may have included theory relating to the grieving process and/or models of communication and counselling. This 'thinking strategies' approach reminds us to consider alternative views and perhaps what did not actually happen. In this situation what Tripp refers to as the 'non events' may also prove valuable to the nurse reflecting on this incident. For example what if this had not gone to plan or if some situation had arisen in the comforting of these parents that made the incident a negative process? In this case the nurse may want to reflect on what might have happened if the named nurse had not been present or if she had been dealing with a child with whom she had not had the opportunity to develop a relationship.

## Critical Incident Analysis used for PREP

As already stated, the PREP requirements ask the practitioner to identify areas and ways of maintaining and continuing their professional development. This can be obtained through learning in and on practice and documented carefully in the ways we are suggesting. It is this practice knowledge that, if recorded and interrogated, can be used for the PREP profile.

### Example 2: Critical Incident Analysis

*Description of incident:*

'On being in charge of the ward as a newly qualified nurse the consultant identified that he and the relatives did not want a patient to be informed of his diagnosis and prognosis. This was a cancer that would mean he had a very poor prognosis. On talking with the patient, with whom I had a good relationship, he asked me if he had cancer as he wanted to sort things out for himself. I did not inform him and he died one week later never being formally told what was wrong. From the time of this conversation our relationship disintegrated as he knew I was withholding information.'

### By whom was it handled?

'The ward round where this information was given was handled by myself and instructions passed onto other shifts.'

### What learning occurred?

'In this situation I felt that my trust was being questioned as conflict occurred between what I had been told by the consultant and relatives and what the patient was asking. For myself, I learnt that although they were attempting to protect the patient he needed to sort himself out and therefore there was a problem with communication between all those involved in his care.'

### What were the outcomes of this incident?

'To listen to all the patient's requests and not to compromise trust and destroy relationships that have been built up. To discuss these issues with all the team and the relatives if the patient is asking for more information as he may have appreciated the truth and prepared himself for a more peaceful death dealing with his affairs and being able to say good bye.'

### How has this incident affected your practice?

'To be more assertive with medical staff and to work as a team keeping them informed of the patient's wishes. To act as a patient's advocate in the giving of information and maintaining their trust.'

## Analysing example 2

Dilemma identification and analysis in this situation is where a conflict of personal values and beliefs over hospital values and beliefs caused some conflict. The analysis of these incidents can identify for the individual their own value system, identify areas of poor or inappropriate practice, where communication is problematic or where patient advocacy may be a potential problem between professionals. The first process here is to identify that a dilemma and conflict of beliefs and/or values is occurring. The next is to analyse why and how to act in the best interests of the clients, colleagues or peers supporting with appropriate professional and/or legislative procedures. In accordance with the nurses', midwives' and health visitors' Code of Professional Conduct (1992) the practitioner must act in the best interest of the individual and observe their own limitations, working collaboratively with other members of the multidisciplinary team. Often some practices can cause personal conflict between what Carper (1978) refers to as our ethical knowledge (see chapter 1) and the values that the institution holds. For example, the institution where an individual works may promote a non smoking policy. The individual however may believe smoking should be permitted for the patients. The conflict caused may result in the nurse experiencing some frustration, but as this can be harmful to colleagues or patients, it must be suppressed and nurses should conform to the policy of the institution. Example 2 used here identifies a dilemma for a newly qualified practitioner in that he is placed in a situation where one health care professional disagrees with his beliefs and he is left to administer the conflicting care prescribed. The inexperience of the newly qualified practitioner may later be used in his PREP profile to identify were he has developed professionally and become more assertive. He may be able to demonstrate an increased ability to justify his actions as he becomes more experienced in dealing with other professionals and those in more senior positions than himself. The situation could equally be used at a job interview to identify how he has learnt through practice and how a change in his practice has occurred through the situation.

## Critical incident analysis for accreditation of prior experiential learning

For accreditation of prior experiential learning (APEL) the individual practitioner is attempting to identify where learning has occurred through their clinical practice and how they can then apply underlying theories to their practice, thus identifying levels of competence. In many situations the APEL procedure may require more analysis of the incident to identify reflection and learning in relation to developing and moving their practice forward. For the APEL process the individual may be asked to present their incident in the form of an essay. For the following example the same format as for the job interview and PREP requirements has been used.

### Example 3: Critical incident analysis

*Description of incident:*

'Over a period of three months the Home was told that we should introduce a model of nursing into our practice. As the charge nurse I put this to the team and it was decided to discuss this and devise our model of nursing that was appropriate to the care we gave. To implement and evaluate this change in practice it actually took the team one year.'

*By whom was it handled?*

'Myself in conjunction with all the members of the Home staff. Management and senior staff were consulted during and after our meetings to approve what was being discussed and to comment on the changes that were being implemented.'

## What learning occurred?

'This proved to be a large area of learning for me as an individual as primarily I had to review all the models available in practice. This involved external visits to other homes to see how they were using them. How to develop a model was then undertaken and the change process was used to incorporate the change successfully.'

## What were the outcomes of this incident?

'As an individual I learnt about the development of nursing models, how to lead a group of practitioners through a process of change and the problems that arise within a group of people with all the negotiation that has to occur between the practitioners and the management structures. It also identified the time it actually took to implement new procedures and the legal implications of such a process.'

## How has this incident affected your practice?

'It has identified the theory and practice of nursing also gaining knowledge concerned with changing practice. The importance of gaining all the teams support when attempting to make such a major change in practice and the importance of evaluating that change.'

### Analysis of example 3

In this situation the 'why' question can be applied to analyse the situation. As discussed in chapter 5, the question 'why' is asked to analyse the underlying values that are held by that practitioner. The analysis of this experience identifies how the individual's practice has developed or may have potentially developed inappropriately. Example 3 could be used as an example where learning has occurred as the practitioner attempts to identify improvements in an area of practice. To deepen the analysis the 'why' challenge could be applied to find out why the change was necessary. Other why-type questions that penetrate deep into this incident might be, 'why did it take a year?' 'why were the senior managers consulted?' 'why were visits to other Homes necessary and so on.

This chapter has attempted to provide the reader with several examples of incidents that can be analysed using a variety of methods. The incident should be written in such a way as to protect individuals and preserve their anonymity. The ethical issues identified in the earlier chapter with regard to journal writing are also pertinent to the writing and sharing of analyses of critical incidents.

# References

Carper, B (1978) Fundemental Patterns of Knowing. *Adv Nurs Sci* **1**: 13–23

Tripp D (1993) *Critical Incidents in Teaching: Developing Critical Judgement*. Routledge, London

UKCC (1990) *The Report of Post Registration Education and Practice Project*. UKCC, London

UKCC (1992) *Professional Code of Conduct*. UKCC, London

# Section C

# Outcomes

# 7

# Implications for practice

The professional journal and the analysis of critical incidents are two processes that facilitate learning. If undertaken systematically and deliberatively they have the potential to impact on practice in three broad ways. We have grouped these under the headings of:

- **The technical**: how the two processes help the health care professional to achieve something concrete and instrumental. In this sense they can be seen as a means to clearly specified ends. Examples of this are fulfilling the PREP requirements, undertaking clinical supervision effectively, addressing the issue of becoming more accountable as stipulated in the Code of Professional Conduct and preparing an APEL claim.

- **The practical**: how the two processes facilitate, nourish and sustain our ability to make wise, competent and ethical decisions and to act compassionately and truly, given the clinical context. Examples of this are clarifying the nature of our professional values, engaging in meaningful dialogues and deepening our understanding of the links between practice and theory.

- **The emancipatory**: how the two learning processes help us to question the status quo, the taken-for-grantedness of our clinical worlds and the historical, social and political forces that serve to liberate and constrain our work. Examples of this are the way the professional journal and the analysis of critical incidents generate nursing knowledge and can help to develop the critically reflective practitioner.

# The Technical

## Post Registration, Education and Practice Requirements (PREP)

PREP came into being in April 1995. Its requirements affect every registered nurse, midwife and health visitor (UKCC, 1990) following their re-registration after this date. In the requirements of PREP the document states that every practitioner must demonstrate their continuing development and how this relates to their clinical competence. This should then be recorded in a personal professional profile (UKCC, 1990). Many practitioners may argue that they have always developed their skills and competence. The difference is that since 1995 everyone will need to 'demonstrate' professional development through the profile. The journal and analysis of critical incidents are valuable sources of evidence of professional development for the individual. Both represent learning accomplishments, future needs and wants. There is no reason why this evidence should not be incorporated into the 'personal professional profile'.

## Undertaking clinical supervision

In the UK government's policy statement 'The Vision for the Future' (DoH, 1993), all health care professionals were being urged to enhance their practice, become competent in self-assessment and develop analytical and reflective skills. The document links this clearly to clinical supervision:

> *'It (clinical supervision) is central to the process of learning and to the expansion of the scope of practice and should be seen as a means of encouraging self-assessment, analytical and reflective skills.'*
>
> (DOH, 1993: 15)

Keeping a professional journal is predicated upon the fact that the practitioner is reflective. Critical incidents become a source of learning for improved clinical action because they require an analysis of practice. Both processes, if done rigorously and systematically over time, can produce reasoned and wise practical knowledge. The practitioner and clinical supervisor can interrogate this knowledge and share insights and experiences with the intention of improving the quality of care given.

## Addressing the Code of Professional Conduct

The nurse, midwife and health visitor's Code of Professional Conduct (UKCC, 1992) states that each practitioner is 'accountable' for their own practice, that they must update their practice, acknowledge their personal limitations and, at all times, be able to justify what they do. This is a big agenda. Justifying practice is about professional accountability. If the professional journal and analysis of critical incidents become true 'companions' for all health carers then the evidence they contain can be used to articulate the different ways practice can be justified. Through both processes strengths are identified, limitations appreciated and action plans formulated.

## Preparing an APEL claim (accreditation of prior experiential learning)

For many, the introduction of the credit accumulation and transfer system (CATS) has added much needed flexibility to learning. At the heart of this system is the module which carries with it a CATS rating, usually in the form of 'points' and at a given 'level'. Points are accumulated upon the successful completion of modules. The points build up towards the specified award. Among other things, modularity, ratings and CATS have opened up the issue of practitioners being accredited, that is being given credit for successful formal study undertaken before entry to the current course (APL — the accreditation of prior learning) and credit for prior experiential learning (APEL). Evidence for the APEL has to be provided by the applicant to the course. The professional journal and the analysis of critical incidents is an excellent source for such evidence of learning from experience.

## The Practical

### Clarifying the nature of our professional values (see Ghaye *et al*, 1996a)

Central to any professional improvement effort is an understanding of the relevance and potency of professional values. Health care is value-based work:

> *'We believe that a fundamental type of knowledge that health care professionals need is what we shall call their "values-based knowledge". The constituents of this knowledge are the caregiver's professional values which give a shape, form and purpose to what they do in their clinical areas. This knowledge is not just linked to practice, but also tied inextricably to — and derived from — that practice. Values-based knowledge informs and constantly transforms practice. The problem is that often we do not know the values we have.'*
> (Ghaye *et al*, 1996: 19)

Knowledge for responsible and competent clinical action is knowledge where value positions, values in action and contradictions between what we say and do are explicit and justified. The processes of journal writing and critical incident analysis can help to bring out into the open the values that make us the kind of health care professional we are.

## Engaging in meaningful dialogues

Dialogues of this kind sustain and nourish organisational cultures for improvement. Dialogues can be with self and/or others. They can raise individual and organisational consciousness. Journal writing and the analysis of critical incidents, as we have depicted them, are personally meaningful dialogues which contain reference to individuals, tasks and a clinical context. The dialogues can be those of:

- **Possibility**: if they reflect not only what was thought and done, but what might have been. In other words that 'which is not yet'

- **Hope**: if they describe, explain and justify how the health care professional tries to bring about relevant, appropriate and ethically grounded improvements in their practice and workplace

- **Confrontation**: if they interrogate practice and avoid celebrating it uncritically

- **Liberation**: as they should contain a discourse about health care couched in a language, and in a form, that is personally created, owned by the writer and not imposed upon them.

## Deepening our understanding of the links between practice and theory (see Ghaye *et al*, 1996b)

In writing this book we have alluded to the fact that we do not believe that it is useful to approach the notions of practice and theory as if they were separate entities which have to be fitted together somehow. We also believe that it is simplistic to think that in fitting things together, some new and wonderful insights and actions will arise, in an almost magical way. Journal entries and critical incidents point up two conceptions of 'practical theory'. The first is that they represent 'theory-as-content'. That is, they both contain content which can be seen as a body of health care knowledge which is known by self, and might usefully be known by others. The second is that they represent 'theory-as-process'. By this we mean that it is through the writing of a professional journal and the analysis of critical incidents that we engage in the process of 'theorising' about our clinical practice. This process reflects an interactive view of practice and theory where ideas guide our thinking and actions and where clinical practice informs and transforms ideas.

> *'Reconstruction of nursing practice and the practice worlds of nurses may occur through this process.'*
> (Cox *et al*, 1991: 378)

## The Emancipatory

What should be clear at this stage is that the professional journal and critical incidents symbolise much more than ways to solve practical problems. They are not merely 'tools' or 'techniques'. This is a truncated definition and misrepresents their full nature and power. We are arguing that they can act as a dynamic source of ideas and actions which have the potential to raise very fundamental questions about the nature of our professionality, how this is understood, how it interacts with practice and generates practical workplace change.

In a very important sense they represent an attempt to discover, understand and then perhaps improve existing patterns and order. This is a vital part of the practitioner's meaning-making process. Accounts of practice often draw upon descriptors such as 'turbulent' and 'chaotic'. Journal writing and critical incident analysis are a commitment to come to know, more deeply and richly, the pattern and order in our clinical work, for we live in a universe of patterns.

'*Every night the stars move in circles across the sky. The seasons cycle at yearly intervals. No two snowflakes are ever exactly the same, but they all have a sixfold symmetry. Tigers and zebras are covered in patterns of stripes, leopards and hyenas are covered in patterns of spots. Intricate trains of waves march across the oceans; very similar trains of sand dunes march across the desert. Coloured arcs of light adorn the sky in the form of rainbows, and a bright circular halo sometimes surrounds the moon on winter nights... Patterns possess utility as well as beauty. Once we have learned to recognise a background pattern, exceptions suddenly stand out. The desert stands still but the lion moves.*'

(Stewart, 1995: 1–3)

Both the professional journal and proformas for the analysis of critical incidents may, at this moment in time, be empty and just waiting for you to make a start. We hope that this book helps you to think through the nature of your commitment to these two learning processes.

'*I have a dream. I am surrounded by — nothing. Not empty space, for there is no space to be empty. Not blackness, for there is nothing to be black. Simply an absence, waiting to become a presence.*'

(Stewart, 1995: vii)

# References

Cox H, Hickson P, Taylor B (1991) Exploring reflection: knowing and constructing practice. In: Gray G, Pratt R (Eds) *Towards a Discipline of Nursing.*Churchill Livingstone, Melbourne

Department of Health (1993) *Vision for the Future.* NHS Management Executive, London

Ghaye T *et al* (1996a) *Professional Values: Being a Professional.* Pentaxion Ltd, Newcastle upon Tyne

Ghaye T *et al* (1996b) *Theory-Practice Relationships: Reconstructing Practice*. Pentaxion Ltd, Newcastle upon Tyne

Stewart I (1995) *Nature's Numbers: Discovering order and pattern in the universe*. Weidenfeld & Nicolson, London

UKCC (1990) *The Report of Post Registration Education and Practice Project*. UKCC, London

UKCC (1992) *Professional Code of Conduct*. UKCC, London

# Conclusion

The topography of health care is a challenging one to understand and navigate our way through. It is a value-laden landscape comprised of different knowledges, power structures and political orientations. It is a dynamic landscape where human relations, opportunities for personal growth and the culture of clinical environments constantly change. It is also a perceptual landscape where health care professionals, clients and their families have differing views and experiences of 'real', 'ideal' and 'expected' quality care. Reflective practice is not only a way of 'reading the map' but provides opportunities to 'transform the map' and to reconfigure it.

This book has had four principle elements to it. First there has been a descriptive element associated with questions like, 'what is reflective practice?', 'what are learning journals and critical incidents?' Secondly, there has been a dialogic element. For example we have said that keeping a learning journal, among other things, gives us the chance to have reflective conversations with self, others and the clinical environment. Critical incident analysis was portrayed as a catalyst for meaningful dialogue between peers, managers, clinical supervisors and so on. Thirdly, the book has contained a critical element. By this we mean that learning through journal writing and the analysis of critical incidents gives us a greater awareness of self as human agent and the politico-economic and socio-historical influences which serve to regulate practice. It is through these two processes that we can question the taken-for-grantedness of our clinical worlds. The process is a potentially destabilising one. This leads us onto the fourth and final element which is an action-oriented one. Just to question things daily does not mean that anything will improve. Action is required. One outcome of reflection is that it should have a consequence. Through reflection-on-action we should come to know the wise, competent and ethical thing to do and have the courage and skills to do and defend it. Through these two learning processes insights, appreciations and commitments to act are enriched and consolidated. The learning which accrues can affirm or challenge why we continue to practice in the way we do.

Throughout the book we have drawn attention to the importance of the 'local', to clinical action in a local context. We have focused on the micro-level where health care professionals observe, experience and influence (to a greater or lesser extent) different forms of domination, resistance, facilitation and commitments to quality care delivery. The content of learning journals and the nature of critical in-cidents often identify when and how care giving situations and health care systems are either sustained or break down. Reflection-on-practice, through these two processes of learn-ing, provides the possibility of generating and implementing strategies for improvement that might actually work.

But we cannot create and enter a better world if we cannot envision and articulate it. The use of learning journals and critical incidents can help us do just this. Both are mediums through which health care professionals create accounts (or 'texts') of what they claim they know and what they want or are able to do with this knowledge of practice-in-context. Each text is often part of a 'tangle-of-texts' (Sumara and Luce-Kapler, 1993), which convey a sense of the tensions, dilemmas and contradictions between the health carer as a human agent, on the one hand, and organisational structures on the other.

Reflection-on-practice, in the ways we have set out in this

book, has the potential to transform our practice and the clinical context in which it takes place. 'All in a day's work' becomes much, much more than habitual, routine and taken-for-granted practice. Learning journals and critical incidents are gateways to a deeper, inner reflection upon ourselves and others, how we wish to be in the world and how we might improve it. In this sense this book aligns itself with a general view of reflective practice that it is a continuing struggle both to:

- Empower the individual through personal and socio-political conscious raising

- Empower groups, and through collective action to build contexts for care that are more just, democratic, compassionate and dignified.

## Reference

Sumara D, Luce-Kapler R (1993) Action research as a writerly text: locating co-labouring in collaboration. *Educational Action Research* **1**: 387–395

# Index